Table of Contents

Copyright © Mometrix Media. You have been licensed one copy of this document for personal use only.
Any other reproduction or redistribution is strictly prohibited. All rights reserved.

Top 20 Test Taking Tips

1. Carefully follow all the test registration procedures
2. Know the test directions, duration, topics, question types, how many questions
3. Setup a flexible study schedule at least 3-4 weeks before test day
4. Study during the time of day you are most alert, relaxed, and stress free
5. Maximize your learning style; visual learner use visual study aids, auditory learner use auditory study aids
6. Focus on your weakest knowledge base
7. Find a study partner to review with and help clarify questions
8. Practice, practice, practice
9. Get a good night's sleep; don't try to cram the night before the test
10. Eat a well balanced meal
11. Know the exact physical location of the testing site; drive the route to the site prior to test day
12. Bring a set of ear plugs; the testing center could be noisy
13. Wear comfortable, loose fitting, layered clothing to the testing center; prepare for it to be either cold or hot during the test
14. Bring at least 2 current forms of ID to the testing center
15. Arrive to the test early; be prepared to wait and be patient
16. Eliminate the obviously wrong answer choices, then guess the first remaining choice
17. Pace yourself; don't rush, but keep working and move on if you get stuck
18. Maintain a positive attitude even if the test is going poorly
19. Keep your first answer unless you are positive it is wrong
20. Check your work, don't make a careless mistake

Copyright © Mometrix Media. You have been licensed one copy of this document for personal use only.
Any other reproduction or redistribution is strictly prohibited. All rights reserved.

Discovery

Discovery tools

- Interrogatories: Written questions submitted to an opposing party, to be answered in writing and under oath. The time period for answers is based upon the rules of the court having jurisdiction.
- Requests for Production of Documents, Things, and Inspections: A written request to produce copies of relevant, nonprivileged documents, including medical records, personal records, or photographs. The time for production is based upon the rules of the court having jurisdiction.
- Requests for Admissions: A written document requesting a party acknowledge or admit certain facts or authenticity of relevant materials. The party must state admittance, denial, or reasons for inability to answer. If not answered within the time required, the requests are considered admitted.
- Physical and Mental Examinations: A physical or mental examination conducted by a neutral physician, normally applicable when the physical or mental condition is an issue of the case (e.g., paternity). The examining physician is chosen by the party requesting the exam, and the LNC will assist in the selection.
- Depositions: Oral examination, under oath before a court reporter, of a person believed to have pertinent knowledge of the facts. All attorneys in the action are invited to attend to question the witness.

Deposition

Purpose of a deposition

The deposition is the sworn testimony of an individual believed to have pertinent information in a lawsuit. The witness, known as a deponent, may not necessarily be a party to the action, but may possess relevant knowledge of the claim. The deposition is recorded by a court reporter, and the witness is under oath during the testimony. The deposition is admissible during trial. The attorneys present are afforded the opportunity to question the witness to ascertain his/her knowledge of the case and, also, determine his/her effectiveness at trial. The deposition of a medical expert may help to avoid the high cost of

Copyright © Mometrix Media. You have been licensed one copy of this document for personal use only. Any other reproduction or redistribution is strictly prohibited. All rights reserved.

his/her testimony at trial. Also, the testimony of the witness is preserved, in the event the witness cannot appear at trial. The witness' testimony may also provide additional avenues of discovery for the plaintiff. The witness may also be able to explain evidence or identify other issues.

Deposition preparation and testimony

The LNC should review all medical records prior to the deposition, as well as relevant information. If the LNC has access to pleadings, review of answers to interrogatories and documents produced by opposing parties will be helpful. If being deposed as an expert, the attorney requesting the LNC's appearance can request production of documents available to, or under the control of, the LNC. However, the LNC should bring to deposition only those materials requested by counsel. The LNC should not volunteer information during testimony, and all answers should be clearly stated for recording by the court reporter. If the LNC does not understand a question, he/she should ask for clarification before answering. The information provided in answers should be only that available or known to the LNC, without the addition of personal opinion. Responses such as "I do not know" or "I do not remember" are appropriate if the LNC is unable to answer the question for these reasons. Basically, the LNC should remain composed and take his/her time to properly answer questions.

Plaintiff and defendant in a lawsuit

The plaintiff is the party who initiates the litigation. This party is the individual claiming damages for injuries caused by another party, the defendant. If the individual who actually suffered the injuries has died, the decedent's next of kin or legal guardian will assume the role of the plaintiff on behalf of the decedent's estate. The defendant is the party (either an individual or a business or other entity) being sued by the plaintiff. The plaintiff alleges that this party caused his/her injuries and damages. In a medical malpractice lawsuit, the defendants may include physicians, nurses, HMOs, insurance companies, hospitals, pharmaceutical companies, or physical therapists.

Copyright © Mometrix Media. You have been licensed one copy of this document for personal use only. Any other reproduction or redistribution is strictly prohibited. All rights reserved.

Prelitigation panel

Before instituting litigation, a state court may require the parties to the action to submit to a prelitigation panel. This panel may be a medical tribunal, medical review panel, or arbitration panel. The panel is designed to determine whether negligence has occurred and will provide an opinion after review and evaluation of the arguments and materials provided by the plaintiff and defendant. Each state maintains its own rules regarding prelitigation panels. Arguments exist to support, as well as negate, the panels. Some defense attorneys argue the panels lessen the possibility of superficial lawsuits. Some plaintiff attorneys argue the panels increase the time involved in the normal legal process, as well as the costs incurred by the parties. In actuality, the panels may delay the litigation process by an estimated 6 to 18 months.

Filing a complaint

The complaint is filed by the plaintiff(s) in a lawsuit. The plaintiff files the complaint with the appropriate court, normally a state court in medical malpractice cases. The complaint contains certain essential elements, which include the names of the plaintiff(s) and defendant(s), the alleged breach of duty or negligence, the damages or injuries suffered by the plaintiff(s), and the request for an award. The specific amount requested to compensate the plaintiff for damages may not necessarily be specified; each state has its own rules regarding this demand. A jury demand may be filed with the complaint as well, which requires that the trial be before a jury. After the complaint has been filed, a sheriff or process server serves the documents upon the defendant(s) named in the complaint, normally by personal service.

<u>Explain the elements of case</u>

Case law research involves searching records on prior court decisions that reflect the basis of the plaintiff's allegations or defendant's defenses. The citation structure contains the case name, citation (decision date, docket number, and court information), a brief summary of the decision, head notes or subject notes, names of the attorneys involved, names of the judges who participated in the decision, names of the judges who did not participate, and the text of the court's opinion. The case law will provide the facts of the action, the issues, discussion regarding each issue and applicable law, the final decision, and the court's reason for arriving at the decision. The researcher must be certain the case

Copyright © Mometrix Media. You have been licensed one copy of this document for personal use only.
Any other reproduction or redistribution is strictly prohibited. All rights reserved.

law is still valid and has not been overturned. Shepard's Case Citations will provide information regarding cases that have been overturned, remanded, or cited in other opinions.

Mediation and arbitration

Both mediation and arbitration may be utilized by the parties to a lawsuit to avoid trial and/or to resolve a conflict sooner than trial might. With mediation, the parties appear before an individual or panel of neutral facilitators. This individual/panel will help the parties reach a conflict resolution agreeable to all parties involved. The mediation is utilized to discuss the issues in an amicable setting, allow the parties to make reasonable decisions, and grant some power over the litigation process. Attorneys, LNCs, judges, health care providers, or social workers may act as mediators. Arbitration is a formal setting, much like the hearings and trial of litigation. In this setting, the parties present discovery and witness lists. The proceeding may be before one arbitrator or a panel. The arbitrator(s) may have the power to award damages, attorney fees, interest, and punitive damages.

Mini-trials

There are two forms of mini-trials. The first form offers a neutral panel of individuals to act as the jury. Other members of the law firm will portray witnesses. An actual judge may or may not be present. The case is presented to the panel as if the attorney were actually participating in the trial. The panel will deliberate as a jury and render a decision. In this form, the panel members can offer suggestions regarding positive and negative testimony and presentation. As a result, the attorney becomes aware of the shortcomings of his/her cause of action. The second form of mini-trial offers attorneys for both sides the opportunity to present each side of the case to the panel. Again, a judge may be present. In this situation, the panel members will not offer suggestions regarding positive and negative aspects of each party's litigation. However, the attorneys are granted a view of how each side's case may proceed in trial.

Copyright © Mometrix Media. You have been licensed one copy of this document for personal use only.
Any other reproduction or redistribution is strictly prohibited. All rights reserved.

Focus groups

Focus groups are normally utilized to help an attorney prepare trial strategy and exhibits. The focus group will review one side of the litigation. This provides the attorney with a view of the positive and negative aspects of the evidence reviewed by group members. When an attorney is aware of these positive and negative points, it may be easier to enter into settlement negotiations. Focus group sessions usually occur in neutral locations and neutral facilitators preside. The facilitators' demeanor should remain neutral throughout the proceeding. They are not normally provided with witness testimony, but receive a summary of expected testimony and a background of the action. The panel then deliberates and renders a decision. The importance of the focus group is not the decision rendered, but the questions facilitators provide to assist with trial and settlement.

Professional negligence intermediate or discovery phase

The LNC should consider the following when evaluating discovery in a professional negligence discovery phase:

- Whether the medical aspects of plaintiff's pleadings have been prepared or the defendant's answers have been submitted. This phase should include interrogatory questions and answers.
- Whether all possible expert witnesses have been determined, including potential conflicts, curriculum vitae review, and fee information. This phase should include the availability of the expert when necessary and the expert's opinion regarding testimony.
- Whether all expert witness reports and opinions have been requested, and if obtained, reviewed for appropriate content.
- Whether the opposing party's expert witnesses and, if possible, reports have been reviewed in detail.
- Whether the client's expert witnesses have been prepared for possible testimony questions, whether deposition or trial. The expert's testimony should be reviewed for potential vulnerabilities.
- Whether all proposed medical exhibits have been reviewed by expert witnesses for recommendations.

Copyright © Mometrix Media. You have been licensed one copy of this document for personal use only. Any other reproduction or redistribution is strictly prohibited. All rights reserved.

Hire-a-judge process

The hire-a-judge process is much like courtroom television programs. This is a form of alternative resolution. The process allows for resolution of an action sooner than can be anticipated if parties await trial. The process involves hiring a retired jurist to hear the testimony and view the evidence. The parties normally divide the cost of the process. Also, the parties will agree to comply with the terms of the judge's decision. This process is similar to arbitration, in that the parties agree prior to the proceeding to comply with the decision and waive the right to appeal. This process can better reflect the courtroom proceeding than focus groups or mini-trials.

Copyright © Mometrix Media. You have been licensed one copy of this document for personal use only. Any other reproduction or redistribution is strictly prohibited. All rights reserved.

Legal Documentation

Purposes for writings by LNCs

The four forms of writing include informative writing, commemorative writing, inquisitive writing, and persuasive writing. Informative writing relays information to the party reading the document. In the case of a LNC, informative writing may include reports, memoranda, chart analyses, literature summaries, and reports evaluating the standard of care. This form should present both sides in a fair, objective manner. Commemorative writing presents a record of the events. Examples include medical chart notations, memoranda documenting conversations, or client intake interviews and conferences with potential experts in summary form. Inquisitive writing is designed to ask questions. This form includes interrogatories and requests to produce (which may require production of documents or an individual). This writing should be detailed to avoid missing information. Persuasive writing is meant to convince an audience of a position. The writings include briefs, motions, and correspondence geared toward settlement. This form of writing should be brief.

Summons and complaint

Purpose and content

The complaint is designed to commence litigation on behalf of a plaintiff. This pleading sets forth the plaintiff's claim(s) against a party (the defendant). The pleading must contain facts that demonstrate a claimant is entitled to damages. The pleading is filed with the court having jurisdiction. The summons is issued by the court taking the complaint. The pleading is prepared by plaintiff's attorney and presented at the time of filing the complaint. The summons is directed to a defendant and informs him/her that litigation has been commenced. The summons also notifies the defendant that he/she has a period of time in which to answer the complaint, and if he/she fails to do so, a default judgment may be entered.

Copyright © Mometrix Media. You have been licensed one copy of this document for personal use only. Any other reproduction or redistribution is strictly prohibited. All rights reserved.

Answer to complaint

The answer is the pleading filed by the defendant. The answer admits or denies the allegations claimed by the plaintiff in the complaint. The answer does not set for specific defenses. The issues in the litigation are joined when the answer is filed with the court and, also, served upon plaintiff's attorney. When issues are joined the parties are aware of the allegations plaintiff must prove. The defendant may allege defenses in the answer, although not required to do so. However, there are certain defenses the defendant may be required to include in the answer and if not done, may suffer waiver of the defense(s). The LNC should be aware of these particular defenses when assisting in preparation of an answer.

Counter-claims, cross-claims, and third-party complaints

Counter-claims are claims that defendant alleges against the plaintiff in the action at issue. The allegations may not necessarily be a result of the plaintiff's alleged claim, the idea being that all issues between the parties would be better resolved in one litigation. The plaintiff must respond to the counter-claim in the same manner as an answer to complaint. A cross-claim is an action by a defendant against another party. The cross-claim is designed to place liability on another defendant. The third-party complaint is filed to add defendants to a lawsuit. The third-party complaint also alleges liability by another party, either wholly or partly.

Legal writing (prewriting, writing, postwriting)

- Prewriting: This is the first step in preparation of effective legal documentation. The party preparing the document should consider the purpose of the document, the party ultimately reading it, and the value of it. The LNC's documents will ordinarily be read by investigators, experts, legal assistants, or attorneys. Since this is an educated audience, the LNC should communicate in a fashion that compliments the readers' abilities.
- Writing: The best way to begin writing a legal document is to outline the role of the document and the necessary contents to fulfill that role. At times, a draft may be an appropriate document for review by an attorney. Then, the formal writing can be prepared utilizing the attorney's notes.
- Postwriting: Once the draft has been prepared, it may be helpful to leave the document for further review for a short period of time (e.g., one day). This can help

Copyright © Mometrix Media. You have been licensed one copy of this document for personal use only. Any other reproduction or redistribution is strictly prohibited. All rights reserved.

the writer review the document with a "fresh eye." Also, the document should be reviewed for organization to be certain each topic is covered in an orderly fashion, headings are correct if used, or graphs are provided if necessary.

Issues to avoid when preparing/writing

The LNC should avoid three forms of language when writing: gender-specific, persuasive, and legalese.

- First, to avoid misinterpretation that can be associated with pronouns, the writer should be clear regarding the person about whom he/she is speaking is a sentence. Generally, the writer should attempt to avoid the use of pronouns.
- Second, the writer should also avoid arguing an issue within the writing. The writing should remain impartial, with the facts stated clearly. The writer should not offer an opinion or judgment regarding whether an action can be won.
- Third, the writer should not use legal phrases such as "to-wit," or "aforementioned." These terms are antiquated and not necessary. To keep the document simple, the writer should not use legal or medical terms, if possible. Also, the parties' names should be used for clarity.

Attributes of reader-friendly writing

Legal documents should be written in an effort to decrease reading time. Information necessary to the document should remain, but unnecessary or repetitive wording should be avoided. The writing should utilize short, simple language. This helps the reader understand the document without consulting a dictionary. Confusion is increased when using long sentences, so short sentences are helpful. The length of paragraphs should also be kept as short as possible. Paragraphs breaks can help keep the reader's attention. Phrases and expressions that do not add to the document should be avoided. The writing should be clearly stated in an effort to avoid multiple meanings or misunderstandings. Simple language should add to the writing's clarity. Last, the writing should be structured. Clear structure helps the reader retain the information and makes reading much easier. Basically, keep the document as simple and short as possible.

Copyright © Mometrix Media. You have been licensed one copy of this document for personal use only. Any other reproduction or redistribution is strictly prohibited. All rights reserved.

Legal correspondence

- Acquiring Information: This type of correspondence requests information such as medical records or litigation updates. The information may be requested from health care providers, employers, insurance companies, or the client.
- Disclosing Information: This type of correspondence communicates information to various parties. The letter may provide the client with an update of the action. A defense attorney may update the insurance company defending the action.
- Confirming Information: This type of correspondence confirms activities that take place prior to, during, and after litigation. A letter may confirm hearing or deposition dates, as well as confirm verbal agreements between parties.
- Rendering an Opinion: This type of correspondence may be used to grant an opinion to a prospective client or offer judgment to an insurance company when a claim is filed.
- Requesting Settlement of a Matter: This type of correspondence is normally prepared by the plaintiff's attorney. This letter summarizes the issues, damages, and plaintiff's request for settlement. This letter attempts to settle an action without trial proceedings.

Settlement brochure

The settlement brochure is normally prepared in addition to the settlement demand letter. Also, the brochure is ordinarily utilized when an action involves intricate or large-scale damages. The brochure supports plaintiff's claim for damages and completely discloses and sets forth the issues, including all reports, evaluations, and expert authority. The settlement brochure may act as an assurance to the insurance company and defense attorney that the plaintiff has confidence in his/her claim. The settlement brochure should contain persuasive text, clearly setting forth the plaintiff's position.

Communication after initial interview

The LNC may be the party involved in the initial interview with a prospective client. Normally, this occurs if the LNC is employed by a referral firm. The LNC must then advise the attorney of the potential client's claim and damages. To that end, the LNC will prepare a memorandum summarizing the interview. The LNC should refer to his/her notes and to

Copyright © Mometrix Media. You have been licensed one copy of this document for personal use only. Any other reproduction or redistribution is strictly prohibited. All rights reserved.

the questionnaire utilized during the interview, if applicable. The LNC should be certain to include all information the attorney will need to properly evaluate the claim. The LNC should also communicate with the client after the interview for the purpose of thanking him/her for the meeting, requesting additional information if necessary, or confirming meetings. Relative to a claim the attorney has accepted, the LNC should be certain to maintain communication with the client on a regular basis.

Correspondence

Correspondence to obtain medical records

The LNC may be responsible for obtaining the medical records of the client. The client must sign a medical release authorization in order to obtain records. The client should sign several forms, although health care providers may accept photocopies. The LNC must be aware of the type of medical authorization necessary to obtain specific records (e.g., AIDS information) that are not within the boundary of ordinary records. The LNC may wish to contact the institution from whom records are to be requested to ascertain fees, if any, and specific information required to obtain the facility's records. The written request should include the client's full name, date of birth, social security number, dates of service, specific records requested, and pre-payment, if possible. If the request is for all records, the LNC should specify emergency room records, radiology reports, etc.

Correspondence to obtain physician and expert reports and records

The LNC may have to obtain a medical reports from a treating physician or a medical expert when the claimant has completed treatment. The LNC should thoroughly review all medical records and client statements prior to requesting a report. The letter to the treating physician should request a detailed prognosis, including symptoms, permanency, or impairment as a result of the injury sustained. The letter to the medical expert should provide all medical records and pertinent information, as well as request a report detailing the expert's opinion regarding medical and legal issues. The expert may act as a witness at trial; if so, the LNC may be required to review correspondence with the expert to assist in determining his/her ability to educate the jury.

Copyright © Mometrix Media. You have been licensed one copy of this document for personal use only. Any other reproduction or redistribution is strictly prohibited. All rights reserved.

The LNC's Role

AALNC Code of Ethics

- The LNC shall not discriminate against any person based upon race, creed, color, age, sex, national origin, social status, or disability and shall not allow personal attitudes to interfere with professional performance.
- The LNC shall perform as a consultant or an expert with the highest degree of integrity.
- The LNC shall use informed judgment, objectivity, and individual competence as the standard for accepting assignments.
- The LNC shall maintain standards of conduct reflecting honorably upon the profession.
- The LNC shall provide professional services with objectivity.
- The LNC shall protect client privacy and confidentiality.
- The LNC shall account for responsibilities accepted and actions performed.
- The LNC shall maintain professional nursing competence.

HMO liability

There are three questions that must be considered when determining whether a managed care action is warranted. The questions will also help assess the claimant's remedies and the manner in which the attorney will plead on behalf of the claimant. The issues to be considered include: (1) whether the claimant sustained meaningful injury; (2) whether the claim will involve an ERISA plan or a non-ERISA/ERISA-exempt entity, as this issue may have a significant bearing upon the cause of action the claimant may plead and the remedies available; and (3) the nature of the managed care entity (e.g., HMO, PPO, traditional indemnity insurance, or point of service contract).

LNC's checklist of issues involved in HMO litigation
When reviewing an HMO action, the LNC normally assists the attorney with determination of whether the promised health care was provided to the claimant. To that end, the LNC should:

Copyright © Mometrix Media. You have been licensed one copy of this document for personal use only. Any other reproduction or redistribution is strictly prohibited. All rights reserved.

- obtain the insurance certificate and all benefit information;
- if a contracted benefit plan was denied by the plan, determine whether the benefit is an industry standard;
- review the summary plan description to determine whether it is understandable;
- determine whether all changes to the plan were made timely with proper notification;
- ascertain that all options available have been attempted (e.g., hearings);
- if all options have not been attempted, determine whether an available option is in the best interest of the member;
- if an emergency exists, determine whether litigation is necessary for immediate relief;
- obtain all documentation detailing the denial;
- research all sources regarding the standard of care for the member's condition, as well as those supporting the claim;
- obtain the opinion of the treating physician;
- determine whether the HMO made a medical decision.

In-house plaintiff LNC

The LNC will normally participate in the initial interview and research to assist the attorney with determination of whether to pursue an action. If the case is rejected, the LNC may prepare the rejection letter for the attorney's signature. If accepted, the LNC will meet with the client a second time to obtain comprehensive information. The LNC will then request medical records, and organize and review the same when received. The LNC will also gather relevant research documentation. After review and research, the LNC will advise the attorney whether or not the action has merit, including possibly preparing a written summary for clarification and reference. The LNC will also assist with obtaining experts. Review with the attorney may occur again after the expert has provided a report. The LNC may assist with pleading preparation, deposition preparation, transcript review, providing relevant information to experts, discovery, and records update throughout litigation.

Copyright © Mometrix Media. You have been licensed one copy of this document for personal use only. Any other reproduction or redistribution is strictly prohibited. All rights reserved.

In-house defendant LNC

The role of the defendant LNC is similar to the role of the plaintiff LNC, with a few exceptions. The LNC will normally become involved in the defense action immediately upon receipt from the insurance carrier or defendant. The LNC will request all medical and other relevant information as soon as the proper authorizations are received from plaintiff's attorney. The LNC will then review the records, research pertinent medical literature and cases, and discuss the action with the defense attorney. The defense LNC may review records specifically relative to preparation for plaintiff's deposition to advise the defense attorney regarding issues affecting liability, causation, damages, or contributory negligence. As with the plaintiff LNC, the defense LNC may assist with pleading preparation, deposition preparation, transcript review, providing relevant information to experts, discovery, and records update throughout litigation.

Roles of the LNC
- Claims consultant/adjuster: The LNC will investigate, evaluate, and negotiate claims, then act as an evaluator, mediator, consultant, or technical analyst.
- Case manager: The LNC will assess claimant needs, then plan and arrange delivery of necessary services and oversee services. The LNC may investigate the claimant's clinical condition and care setting, as well as the patient's progress.
- Benefits coordinator: The LNC will understand, interpret, analyze, and calculate the benefits available to the claimant, as well as ascertain the benefits will meet the claimant's needs.
- Workers' compensation manager: The LNC will determine the needs of the claimant, as well as plan and monitor the services required by the claimant. Medical policy coordinator: The LNC may create or amend medical policies when necessary or requested by the insurance company. Utilization review coordinator: The LNC will determine the claimant's medical need and the suitability for the claimant's benefit use.
- Risk manager: The LNC will investigate and institute policies to reduce claim damages and loss.
- Medical malpractice/liability consultant: The LNC will participate in an initial claim to obtain and review client records and interviews, provide information to the

- 18 -

Copyright © Mometrix Media. You have been licensed one copy of this document for personal use only. Any other reproduction or redistribution is strictly prohibited. All rights reserved.

attorney, and assist with experts and clinical research. Then, the LNC will continue to participate in the action as it progresses.

Credentials and certifications

- Certified Disability Management Specialist (CDMS): A nonprofessional certificate, the certification is acquired through examination plus two years experience working with the disabled population in the disability-compensation system.
- Certified Registered Rehabilitation Nurse (CRRN): A professional certificate, the certification is available only to registered nurses through the Association of Rehabilitation Nurses. The certificate is acquired through examination and two years experience working in rehabilitation.
- Certified Rehabilitation Counselor (CRC): A professional certificate, the certification is available to master's-prepared rehabilitation counselors and acquired through examination and demonstrated work experience.
- Certified Case Manager (CCM): A professional certificate, this certification is acquired through demonstration of two or more years' experience in case management.

Copyright © Mometrix Media. You have been licensed one copy of this document for personal use only. Any other reproduction or redistribution is strictly prohibited. All rights reserved.

Medical Malpractice

LNC's role prior to deposition of a medical expert

The LNC's role prior to the deposition is to assist in preparation. The LNC must review medical records to identify areas of failure in standards of care, especially when related to the deponent. The LNC will prepare questions relative to medical practices and issues. Reviewing answers to interrogatories and medical records will help the LNC prepare questions and explain information that may be confusing for the attorney. The LNC must obtain all information available about the deponent. This information may include the curriculum vitae, licensing records, and disciplinary action. The LNC should review the applicable state court records to determine whether the witness has been a defendant in previous actions. If found, the LNC should obtain relevant records from the previous litigation to review prior to deposition. A search for all articles or other writings by the witness will be helpful, particularly those relative to the lawsuit. All writings should be summarized for the attorney, especially noting discrepancies between the witness' viewpoint in the writing versus his/her view in the case being reviewed.

LNC's role in triaging a medical malpractice claim

The LNC reviews the elements of triage to assist the attorney in determining whether a claim on behalf of a client exists. The review includes elements of liability, damage, causation, statute of limitations, contributory/comparative negligence, conflict of interest, economics, defendants, the client, venue and jurisdiction, informed consent, cosmetic surgery cases, previous rejection of the case, and cooperation of subsequent treating physicians. A registered nurse possesses the ability to properly focus on the merits or problems of a potential lawsuit. To pursue the claim, many of the above elements must be present; one or two elements are not enough to justify litigation. Although the attorney will make the final decision regarding the claim, the LNC must advise him/her of potential problems. Also, most malpractice claims are taken on a contingency basis, which means the attorney will not be paid if damages are not awarded to his/her client. The LNC's advice regarding problems with the elements of triage becomes important to avoid this loss.

Copyright © Mometrix Media. You have been licensed one copy of this document for personal use only.
Any other reproduction or redistribution is strictly prohibited. All rights reserved.

LNC's investigation of medical malpractice liability

Also known as negligence, liability must be determined before an attorney will proceed on behalf of a client. The LNC should consider not only the plaintiff's reasons for negligence, but also thoroughly review the records. The records review may reveal that the actions taken were acceptable or that the actual negligence is different than the plaintiff believes. The LNC should consider several questions during case review, including the actions of the health care provider and the accepted standards of practice, whether a reasonable practitioner in the same situation would have performed similar actions, or whether the complications were common. When reviewing records, the LNC must keep in mind that the liability must be based upon the information available to the health care provider at the time and place in question. If the LNC is unable to determine liability after review of the records and information available, the LNC should presume liability exists.

Damages in medical malpractice cases

Special, general, and punitive represent the three types of damages.
- Special damages consist of out-of-pocket expenses the claimant incurred as a result of the alleged negligence.
- General damages are non-monetary damages that have a value for which plaintiff should be compensated, but damages upon which the law is unable to place a dollar value. Pain and suffering is an example of general damages.
- Punitive damages are those that exceed the amount intended to properly compensate the claimant.

These damages are also known as exemplary damages. The purpose of punitive damages is to punish a defendant, set an example, and discourage inappropriate behavior in the future. The LNC must review all aspects of the claimant's life and the impact the injury has had upon the claimant, including the ability to work, physical activity, and permanent impairment. The plaintiff's health history should also be reviewed, as pre-existing conditions, surgeries, medical bills, and disability that plaintiff would have suffered regardless of the standard of care cannot be claimed as damages.

Copyright © Mometrix Media. You have been licensed one copy of this document for personal use only.
Any other reproduction or redistribution is strictly prohibited. All rights reserved.

Theory of recovery

The theory of recovery for a patient's loss of chance of survival or loss of chance of a better recovery is recognized under certain jurisdictions. In this instance, the physical harm as a result of an initial condition is not the injury for which the claimant is compensated. The claimant's lost chance at attaining a better result is the actual injury subject to compensation. The theory is employed when a plaintiff has a pre-existing injury or illness which worsens as a result of the alleged negligence of the defendant resulting in the patient's death when a significant chance of survival might have existed without the negligence or the patient might have survived the illness if there had been no delay in diagnosis. In some jurisdictions, the plaintiff's claim may be affected by the actual chance of survival when the alleged negligence occurred. For instance, if plaintiff had a less than 50% chance of survival at the time of negligence, no claim for negligence would exist.

Reviewing causation in medical malpractice case

The negligence claimed by plaintiff must be causally related to the actual injury claimed by plaintiff. To that end, the LNC must consider several questions: (1) whether the negligence caused the injury, (2) whether the negligence might have been responsible for only part of the injury/damages, (3) whether the negligence caused all of the damages, (4) if the negligence did not cause all damages, which part did the negligence actually cause, or (5) would the plaintiff's result have been different if the negligence had not occurred. The LNC must determine the damages suffered by the claimant as a result of the negligence and those suffered regardless of the alleged negligence. The LNC should consult the jury instruction guides for the particular state in which the claim is based to confirm the actual definition of cause.

Statute of limitations in medical malpractice claims

The state having jurisdiction determines the statute of limitations for medical malpractice claims. Most states' statute of limitations is three years, but the determination of the actual date may be affected by several factors. In a breach of contract or breach of promise or warranty action, the statute may be six years. Also, the statute may affect minors or mentally impaired individuals differently, as well as death claims and time lapses between discovery of the injury or negligence. For intentional tort claims (e.g., assault, battery), the

Copyright © Mometrix Media. You have been licensed one copy of this document for personal use only. Any other reproduction or redistribution is strictly prohibited. All rights reserved.

statute is normally two years. In most instances, the date of the actual wrongdoing normally determines the beginning of the limitations period. However, since the negligence might not be evident at the time the negligence occurred, many states allow the period to begin upon discovery of the injury or the date when it should have been reasonably discovered. With wrongful death, the statute may begin to run upon date of death, although this is not the case in every situation. The LNC should review the medical records to determine dates that affect the statute of limitations.

Contributory negligence and comparative negligence

Contributory negligence has been terminated in many states. In states recognizing this defense, contributory negligence totally bars a claimant's recovery when the plaintiff is found to have contributed to any of the damages suffered. Contributory negligence normally occurs when a patient fails to follow prescribed treatment or fails to follow up as recommended. Also, the plaintiff may be subject to contributory negligence if he/she lies about his/her condition or withholds information from the health care provider. Further, contributory negligence cannot be utilized as a defense in claims based upon lack of informed consent. Most states recognize comparative negligence which determines the plaintiff's portion of contribution to the damages or injuries claimed. In the case of comparative negligence, the award is based upon a percentage of fault to the plaintiff, and that amount is deducted from the amount due to plaintiff. When reviewing records, the LNC should consider whether the plaintiff contributed to the injuries or damages in any manner.

Conflict of interest

The LNC should, as soon as possible, make every effort to determine if conflicts exist. The client's best interest is the goal of the LNC, and a conflict of interest will be detrimental to achieving that goal. The ABA Model Rules of Professional Conduct, Rule 1.7, "General Rule of Conflict of Interest," states that no issue should be undertaken if any issue or knowledge exists that would be "directly adverse to another client." Thus, the LNC must be aware of all clients when investigating a possible claim. Also, Rule 1.9 of the ABA Model Rules of Professional Conduct provides that a conflict of interest exists when an action can be "materially adverse to the interests of the former client unless the former client consents after consultation." Other areas of conflict that may arise include an LNC working for both

Copyright © Mometrix Media. You have been licensed one copy of this document for personal use only. Any other reproduction or redistribution is strictly prohibited. All rights reserved.

a plaintiff and defendant in an action, changing from one side to another during an action, cases in which the health care providers are known to the LNC personally, and cases involving parties known or related to the LNC. The LNC must inform the attorney if he/she believes a conflict of interest exists.

Economic factors

Most attorneys will not pursue claims with a value less than $150,000. On average, pursuit of a claim will cost from $25,000 to $100,000 in out-of-pocket expenses and time. The LNC should review the records with regard to the value of the claim versus the time and expenses involved in litigation. In addition, sovereign immunity must be considered. Some institutions, providers, and governmental agencies are afforded protection from liability and, in fact, there may be limits set regarding liability. Also, an action involving vaccines or brain-damaged babies may be subject to a compensation fund governed by state or federal laws, which funds may have liability limits as well.

Representation of the client

The LNC will make observations when first meeting a client. Those observations will include various factors regarding the client's viability as a claimant. The LNC will help determine how the jury will perceive the client if he/she appears in court. The LNC should be aware of several issues that may pose a problem with the client. An issue of credibility may arise in the event the client makes a statement conflicting with the record. A client may be regarded as dishonest by a jury based upon appearance or because of a questionable background. A criminal record may have a negative impact with a jury. A disagreeable appearance or dubious job may alter a jury's perception. A jury may look unfavorably upon a client with a background involving drugs, abuse, or alcoholism. Greedy clients can be discerned by judges and juries. Last, any indication that the client may not cooperate fully with the attorney during litigation (answering interrogatories, appearing for hearings, producing documents, etc.) will be a negative issue during representation.

Role of the LNC in the medical malpractice claims arena

The LNC will provide medical expertise, a network of professional contacts, analysis and evaluation of records and information, and access to medical literature helpful to claims.

Copyright © Mometrix Media. You have been licensed one copy of this document for personal use only. Any other reproduction or redistribution is strictly prohibited. All rights reserved.

The LNC's medical experience will assist in review, summary, and evaluation of medical records. The LNC's experience also aids in locating gaps or missing records and information. Damages can be assessed, especially in the area of medical damages, and evaluation of medical records can be performed to confirm the necessity and relevance of all treatments. In the event an expert medical witness is required, the LNC can assist in compilation of the information provided to the expert for preparation of examination and/or testimony. The LNC may prepare summaries and analysis for the attorney. While the action is pending, the LNC may be called upon to draft or respond to medical discovery, attend independent medical examinations, work with team members to prepare visual aids and exhibits, attend and assist with depositions, or attend and assist at trial.

Defenses to medical negligence

- Failure to Take Precautions to Minimize Damages: The plaintiff must take appropriate measures to minimize or negate possible injury. For example, failure to wear a seat belt may contribute to injury, resulting in plaintiff's failure to take appropriate precautions.
- Errors of Judgment: If a health care provider exercised reasonable care in the treatment of a patient, but the treatment prescribed failed, the health care provider is not liable for injuries or damages that result. The health care provider must have exercised essential skill, care, and knowledge when treating a patient.
- Employment Retirement Income Security Act: Health maintenance organizations managed and owned by employees for the benefit of employees and their families may be exempt from liability under the Employment Retirement Income Security Act (ERISA) of 1974.
- Constitutional Defenses: The Ninth Amendment of the United States Constitution protects people's natural rights whether enumerated therein or not. One of these rights is the patient's right to refuse or accept treatment.
- Charitable Immunity: Although limited in some states and abolished in most, this defense restricts liability to religious, educational, and nonprofit organizations organized for charitable purposes.

Copyright © Mometrix Media. You have been licensed one copy of this document for personal use only. Any other reproduction or redistribution is strictly prohibited. All rights reserved.

Definitions

- Vicarious Liability: The imposition of liability on one party for the acts or omissions of another party. Thus, a nurse acting under the direction of a physician may be found negligent.

- Borrowed Servants: Employees loaned to another party for a particular purpose. Pursuant to this rule, a nurse employed by a hospital, but acting under the direction of a physician not employed by the hospital, is not responsible for negligence (the physician is responsible).

- Res Ipsa Loquitor: "The thing speaks for itself." The facts support the claim of negligence, such as a surgeon operating on the wrong patient.

- Quasi Contract: An implied contract designed to obstruct unjust enrichment. For example, this contract exists to provide emergency treatment for an unconscious patient.

- Hedonic Damages: Damages awarded in the case of a party's loss of enjoyment of life. These damages are also referred to as holistic damages.

- Bylaws: Rules adopted by a health care facility to govern practice relative to medical, surgical, and nurse personnel are referred to as bylaws. The bylaws may extend beyond standards of practice to include credential requirements and conduct.

- Policy: Policies of a health care facility represent the overall program designed to accomplish goals. Policies may be broad in scope and affect several services or departments.

- Procedures: Procedures encompass the programs or steps taken to carry out the health care facility's policies.

- Relevant: Relevance, in general, pertains to evidence utilized to prove or disprove an issue. When utilized in standards of care, the evidence must be relevant to factual issues of the litigation. In this respect, the evidence must pertain not only to the subject, but the time in question.

- Hearsay evidence: If a witness does not personally testify regarding the validity of evidence, the evidence may be considered hearsay evidence. Relative to standards of care, evidence may be considered hearsay if the author to a document pertaining to standards is not present as a witness.

Copyright © Mometrix Media. You have been licensed one copy of this document for personal use only. Any other reproduction or redistribution is strictly prohibited. All rights reserved.

- Error-in-judgment rule: Relative to standards of care, this defense to malpractice provides that the health care provider met the standard of care despite the fact that an error occurred.
- Two-schools-of-thought-doctrine: Relative to standards of care, this defense to malpractice provides that a health care provider is not negligent when one of several recognized, available treatment methods is adopted.
-

Good Samaritan laws

Individuals who provide medical assistance at an accident scene, emergency, or disaster are protected pursuant to Good Samaritan laws. Health care providers who utilize accepted standards of care when offering assistance are normally covered under these laws. However, the laws will not protect health care providers who are negligent during the course of employment. The Good Samaritan laws cannot be used as a defense if the provider receives a fee for services. The laws cannot be invoked if the person receiving care is intentionally harmed or gross negligence is found to exist. The laws may relate to nurses and physicians in a different manner from state to state.

Jury selection procedure

The jury selection will take place on the first day of the jury trial. The selection will be from a pool of citizens from the area of the jurisdictional court. The potential jurors will be asked questions by the judge or the attorneys for the plaintiff and defendant in the action. The questions will be designed to determine prejudices, biases, or any relationship between the plaintiffs, defendants, attorneys, or significant others and the juror. The process is known as voir dire. Each attorney may invoke peremptory challenges or present a challenge for cause relative to a potential juror. The peremptory challenge will eliminate a potential juror without cause shown for his/her removal. If an attorney cites bias or prejudice for removal of a potential juror, the juror will be dismissed as a result of a "challenge for cause." Malpractice actions normally involve 12 jurors, with one or two alternates.

Copyright © Mometrix Media. You have been licensed one copy of this document for personal use only.
Any other reproduction or redistribution is strictly prohibited. All rights reserved.

Standards of care

- Standards of professional performance: This performance reflects activities such as research, ethics, peer review, or education. The performance relates to competency, as opposed to reasonable care or a specific performance level.
- Standard: A standard reflects an authoritative method of care to be followed. Standards do not command conformity to recommended guidelines.
- Guideline: Unlike a standard, a guideline proposes procedures or policies to effect standards of care.

Generally accepted concepts

- Licensing regulations: A health care provider should hold a required license to practice pursuant to minimum standards for education and experience; failure is considered prima facie evidence of negligence.
- State Laws and Administrative Regulations: A health care provider is required to meet statutory requirements for standard of care; failure may be deemed negligence.
- Policies and procedures: A health care provider must follow the policies and procedures established by the facility; failure may result in proof of lack of appropriate care.
- Tort law: Case law provides standards of care and liability; failure to meet the standards may be deemed failure to provide appropriate care.
- Scope of practice: Many health care specialties outline the scope of a health care provider's practice, identifying the care that should have resulted.
- Manuals, textbooks, and treatises: Operation manuals provide standards of care relative to medical devices. Textbooks can be utilized to confirm procedures for reasonable care in a given situation. Treatises can establish a standard of care if a health care provider is deemed an expert in a particular field.
- Joint Commission on Accreditation of Healthcare Organizations: The standards provided by the JCAHO are normally accepted nationwide.

Standards of care liability

- Duty: The LNC may need to review whether there was a health care provider duty to perform specific functions on behalf of a patient. The LNC should review the nature of the relationship between the health care provider and the claimant.

Copyright © Mometrix Media. You have been licensed one copy of this document for personal use only. Any other reproduction or redistribution is strictly prohibited. All rights reserved.

- Breach/Negligence: The LNC should review the record to determine whether the health care provider failed to meet the standards of care generally accepted, or whether the health care provider performed treatment that a reasonable health care provider would not perform in the same situation.
- Damages: The claimant must have sustained an injury. The medical damages can result from financial, physical, or emotional injury.
- Proximate cause: The claimant's damages must be a direct result of, or caused by, the negligent act(s) of the health care provider.

Copyright © Mometrix Media. You have been licensed one copy of this document for personal use only. Any other reproduction or redistribution is strictly prohibited. All rights reserved.

Personal Injury

Purpose of personal injury litigation

Personal injury litigation serves to compensate an individual or individuals for injuries sustained as a result of another's wrongful actions. It encourages individuals to act responsibly and safely, as well as placing liability upon those individuals with the most control over circumstances. It also distributes risk among the liability insurance system. There are several incidents that may result in injury, including transportation incidents (particularly motor vehicle collisions), premises liability (falls, escalator accidents), workplace accidents, product liability cases resulting from defective products, or animals or toxic substances incidents. The law of torts is used in personal injury litigation. In general, any incident or occurrence that results in an injury may lead to a personal injury lawsuit.

Plaintiff's and defendant's elements in proving tort in personal injury actions

Each type of tort maintains certain elements to prove a cause of action exists. Also, each type has defenses that can be used to refute claims. A burden of proof must be shown by the plaintiff's attorney, which requires he/she put forth evidence sufficient to satisfy each element of the tort upon which the lawsuit is based. The preponderance of the evidence standard is the burden of proof in a tort action, requiring that plaintiff demonstrate "it is more probable than not." Normally, a party must show that over 50% of the evidence supports the claim. On the other hand, the defendant's attorney must refute at least one of the elements of the claimant's burden of proof. Affirmative defenses may also be presented by defendant's attorney, but in this case, the defendant's attorney assumes the burden of proof. Most personal injury actions fall under the tort of negligence. In a negligence action, the plaintiff asserts that the defendant failed to exercise reasonable care or caution that resulted in plaintiff's injuries.

Copyright © Mometrix Media. You have been licensed one copy of this document for personal use only.
Any other reproduction or redistribution is strictly prohibited. All rights reserved.

Elements of negligence in a personal injury action

First, the failure to use reasonable care in a situation or circumstance is the liability element of negligence. In reviewing records, the LNC should question whether an alleged defendant failed to exercise reasonable care in a given situation, and if so, the party who is actually liable for the injury. Medical records may disclose this information. Second, the LNC or attorney must determine whether the failure of the alleged defendant caused the injury or damages to plaintiff. A question to be answered in this instance might be whether the failure was a considerable factor in the cause of the injury. In the case of a physical injury, the LNC should review the medical records to help determine which injuries were a result of pre-existing conditions and which were the result of the incident in question. Third, the LNC or attorney must determine whether harm resulted from the actions of defendant. The damages can be established using both the billing records and the medical records.

Damages encountered in a personal injury action

- Special damages: These include the out-of-pocket costs for medical care related to the incident, including the care received at the time of the incident, during litigation, and future care. These costs can include medications, home care services, travel costs for medical treatment. Wage loss can also be a special damage. Under the collateral source rule, the defendant's attorney cannot inform the jury that plaintiff had health insurance coverage.
- General damages: The monetary award for this type of damage is based upon severity of damages and impact on plaintiff's life. These damages may include pain and suffering, fear, or embarrassment.
- Punitive Damages: These are also known as exemplary damages. The plaintiff may receive these damages if defendant is determined to be oppressive, fraudulent, or malicious in behavior. Each state may maintain its own rules for awarding punitive damages.
- Loss of Consortium: This claim can be made by the spouse of a claimant. Basically, this is an assertion of claims such as loss of love, companionship, sexual relations, or home maintenance.

Copyright © Mometrix Media. You have been licensed one copy of this document for personal use only. Any other reproduction or redistribution is strictly prohibited. All rights reserved.

Personal injury action settlement

Ordinarily, the party found liable for injuries has insurance coverage that pays for damages awarded. In the case of an automobile accident, the award or settlement is paid by the insurance company of the party found liable. Although the liable parties may be a vehicle owner and driver of the vehicle, the insurance company that will pay the award is the owner's policy. Payment in premises liability cases will be through the property owner's insurance carrier or the commercial general liability policy in the case of a business. Some policies may contain clauses that cover losses above a certain amount, known as excess coverage. Insurance companies pledge both defense and payment of awards on behalf of the insured party in exchange for payment of premiums by the party. The insurance company will choose the attorney defending the action and normally oversee defense of the litigation. The defendant has a duty to cooperate with the insurance carrier and the defense attorney chosen on his/her behalf.

Insurance coverages/non-coverages

- Uninsured/underinsured coverage: A driver or passengers injured by another driver who is uninsured or underinsured may receive payment through the driver's insurance company. Uninsured motorist coverage is enacted when a liable driver maintains no insurance coverage. Underinsured coverage applies when the policy limits of a liable driver are not sufficient to cover damages awarded.
- Lack of insurance: If a liable driver does not have valid insurance coverage at the time of an accident, he/she may be required to pay an award from personal assets.
- Self-insured entities: A hospital, university, or other large business entity may choose to self-insure by maintaining a fund to cover defense costs and damage awards.
- No-fault insurance: Under this system, each party's insurance coverage pays damages for its insured, whether or not its insured is at fault. However, an injured party is entitled to sue for non-economic losses in certain situations determined by state law and policy coverage. Thirteen states have enacted this system.

Defenses to negligence in personal injury actions

- Comparative negligence: An alleged defendant claims that the plaintiff caused his/her own injury. Each state maintains its own rules regarding comparative

Copyright © Mometrix Media. You have been licensed one copy of this document for personal use only. Any other reproduction or redistribution is strictly prohibited. All rights reserved.

negligence. Normally, the award will be decreased proportionately to the percent of the negligence attributable to plaintiff.

- Seat belt defense: This is a form of comparative negligence, wherein the plaintiff was not wearing a seat belt at the time of the accident. In this instance, the defense attorney will determine the amount of damages the claimant would have sustained if he/she had been wearing the seat belt.
- Assumption of risk: In this instance, the claimant assumes the risk of participating in the activity causing the injury or damages. Recreational activities that cannot be made safe without significantly changing the activity fall within the scope of assumption of risk.

Definitions

- Insurance: A contract provided to a party to cover services, injuries, or damages; the contract will designate conditions, types, and terms of coverage.
- Insurer: A party that agrees to reimburse a second party for loss incurred pursuant to contingencies designated by the first party.
- Collateral source rule: A rule that prohibits a defendant from disclosing to a jury that a plaintiff maintained health insurance coverage to pay all or part of damages.
- Judgment proof: A term used to describe an action when no significant assets are available to satisfy a judgment.
- PIP: Personal Injury Protection – Coverage provided by a party's automobile insurance for his/her medical expenses incurred in the event of an accident.

Liability experts and causation experts

- Forensic anatomist: This expert reviews causation of the injury, including mechanism of the injury, anatomy of the claimant, radiology/imaging studies information, clinical data, and surgical findings.
- Biomechanical/biomedical engineer: This expert review collision information to calculate data regarding forces. He/she may inspect the vehicle and scene of the accident.
- Human factors engineer: This expert reviews people's interaction with their surroundings. He/she may be called upon in the event of alleged human error.
- Physicians: This expert may conduct an independent medical examination regarding alleged injuries, as well as causation findings.

Copyright © Mometrix Media. You have been licensed one copy of this document for personal use only. Any other reproduction or redistribution is strictly prohibited. All rights reserved.

- Forensic pathologist: In a wrongful death claim, this expert offers judgment about the cause of death. He/she may offer an opinion regarding the specific cause of death in the event of many injuries.

Damage experts
- Vocational experts: This expert renders an opinion regarding the claimant's ability to perform his/her specific job functions. He/she may also offer an opinion regarding the degree of impairment and whether vocational rehabilitation is required if the claimant cannot return to work.
- Life care planning expert: This expert is normally a nurse who has training in this area. This expert can determine future needs and the cost of those needs, including changes to a claimant's home.
- Economist: This expert calculates damages, including future medical costs, inflation adjustment, and likely future income loss.
- Life expectancy experts: This expert may be an actuary, Ph.D., or medical doctor. He/she offers judgment relative to claimant's life expectancy.

LNC's role in analyzing medical records

The LNC's role in reviewing medical records may be on behalf of a plaintiff or a defendant in litigation. The review should focus on identification of issues in the action, strengths and weaknesses of the issues, and additional evidence the LNC deems important. The LNC does not review the records as an expert in the areas of biomechanics or causation. Rather, the LNC performs issue-spotting, fact identification to determine appropriate liability of any parties, inconsistencies between the claimant's complaints and the findings in the records, and opinions regarding consistency between the claimed injuries and those documented requiring additional discovery. The LNC should also be aware of possible missing records, identifying each, if possible.

Reviewing medical records

The LNC should note agreement or disagreement between the claimant's description of the accident and injuries, as well as his/her idea of the injuries' cause. The claimant's statements, especially relative to another party's possible liability, should be noted. The

Copyright © Mometrix Media. You have been licensed one copy of this document for personal use only. Any other reproduction or redistribution is strictly prohibited. All rights reserved.

medical records should be reviewed alongside discovery documents to confirm accuracy. The LNC should be wary of plaintiff's injury descriptions when too accurate. Plaintiff's pre-existing conditions should be noted, especially as they relate to plaintiff's claim. The LNC should note when plaintiff delayed seeking treatment or for treatment gaps, including failure to comply with prescribed treatment. Injuries sustained after the accident should be noted. Also, the LNC should register when a health care provider has expressed doubts in any medical record. The plaintiff's normal activities (including those involving his/her relationship with a spouse) should be reviewed to confirm he/she is operating within the limits of the injuries or that limitations in normal activity confirm the injury. The plaintiff's emotional health is an issue to be observed.

Educating attorney

The LNC can provide information about medical conditions, anatomy, and physiology in a manner understandable by the attorney. The LNC can also enlighten the attorney regarding the plaintiff's claimed injuries. The pronunciation of medical terminology is sometimes difficult, so assisting the attorney in this area is essential. In order to effectively discuss the litigation with opposing attorneys, adjusters, or medical experts, the attorney must be able to pronounce pertinent medical terms and understand those terms when referring to plaintiff's injuries. The attorney will also benefit from teaching materials to review the medical information. These materials may include books, articles, drawings, diagrams, websites, computer programs, or companies that provide medical educational guides.

Organizing medical records

The LNC will not only review the medical records, but will organize the records for the attorney's review. One manner of organization is chronological. To thoroughly organize the information in chronological fashion, a summary of each visit, procedure, diagnostic test, and additional entries should be noted by date. After chronological organization, a narrative should be prepared. Obviously, the chronology will assist in preparation of this format. The chronological and narrative record can then be compared to assist in noting missing records, essential issues, and positive and negative medical aspects of the claim.

Copyright © Mometrix Media. You have been licensed one copy of this document for personal use only. Any other reproduction or redistribution is strictly prohibited. All rights reserved.

Searching medical literature for an attorney

The LNC should review and search relevant medical literature to assist the attorney to understand the claimant's medical issues, to effectively discuss the injuries with opposing parties and medical experts, and for preparation of litigation. The search will assist the attorney in determining causation and damages. Relative to damages, medical research will assist in determination of not only current, but long-term issues faced by the plaintiff. This information can be used by the attorney in settlement demands and discussions with opposing parties. Peer-reviewed medical literature websites include the PubMed/MEDLINE database and MD Consult.

Assistance with discovery

The LNC's review of the medical records will assist the attorney when preparing discovery documentation or scheduling depositions and witness testimony. Review of medical records will help the LNC determine additional records needed to accurately determine injuries and damages. Those records can then be included in discovery documents, such as requests for production and interrogatories. Also, the records review may disclose additional physicians or medical institutions from which records should be obtained. The LNC may also determine additional records are required after review of the accident report or employment record. After review of all records, the LNC will be able to suggest questions to be included in interrogatories or utilized at depositions.

Assisting with personal injury settlement document preparation

The LNC's review of medical and other records will allow him/her to help the attorney draft settlement documents. The demand letter sent to the insurance adjuster before litigation is filed itemizes the insured party's liability and the injuries of the claimant. Because of records review, the LNC is able to interpret and summarize vital information for the attorney to include in a demand letter. This information can coax the insurance company to settle the claim. The LNC can offer suggestions for exhibits, as well as calculate the costs of medical care. These items are helpful when included in a demand letter. If the claim proceeds to a lawsuit, the attorney may prepare a settlement package for the insurance company's consideration. The LNC can assist in preparation of this package, which will likely include more detailed information than a demand letter. These settlement

Copyright © Mometrix Media. You have been licensed one copy of this document for personal use only. Any other reproduction or redistribution is strictly prohibited. All rights reserved.

documents must illustrate the claimant's injuries and damages effectively, and the LNC should offer suggestions that accomplish this task.

Expert fact witness and locating expert witnesses

The LNC may act as an expert fact witness based upon his/her clinical experience and knowledge. In this role, the LNC will review the medical records and literature pertinent to the claimant's action. The LNC will utilize this information to testify before a jury. In this role, the LNC will explain the factual material in layperson's terms. Since the LNC does not offer judgment regarding standard of care, his/her testimony can be effective in a personal injury action. The LNC is able to turn volumes of medical information into understandable format for the attorney and the jury. The LNC can also act as a defense expert fact witness when refuting the plaintiff's injury claim. If not acting as a witness, the LNC may be called upon to locate an expert witness. In this instance, the LNC may locate not only medical experts, but accident reconstructionists, economists, or biomechanical engineers. To that end, the LNC should gather information regarding these expert witnesses and their expected ability to testify to issues essential to the attorney's case.

LNC's role in trial preparation

One way to assist the attorney in trial preparation is to create or obtain evidence that will effectively demonstrate the claims of plaintiff. The jury should be able to understand and associate with the illustrations presented. All entries in the medical records that are important to the case should be reviewed and, if applicable, copied or "blown up" for juror inspection. The LNC should obtain and prepare all exhibits in an effort to make each understandable and clear to the jury, as well as allow them to make an educated decision. Review of the deposition and other discovery documents prior to trial will allow the LNC to suggest questions to be asked of witnesses. In addition, the LNC's compilation of trial documents and information may disclose issues that should be addressed prior to or during trial.

Kinematics and impact location

Occupant kinematics involves the movement of occupants in a motor vehicle due to the impact of the collision. The LNC who has knowledge of occupant kinematics can more

Copyright © Mometrix Media. You have been licensed one copy of this document for personal use only. Any other reproduction or redistribution is strictly prohibited. All rights reserved.

effectively analyze the medical records. Also, the LNC can better imagine the collision with knowledge of biomechanics and occupant kinematics. However, a serious collision will likely require the skills of an accident reconstructionist. This expert will review the facts of the accident and make a determination regarding the load on the occupants. The LNC should obtain a copy of any reports of accident reconstructionists. Also, the LNC should have some knowledge of description used in the report, including the location of vehicles. The numbers on the clock are utilized for this purpose. The vehicle in the center is facing toward the 12, and all other vehicles involved surround that vehicle. The straight-on frontal collision is described as 12 o'clock, and the straight-on rear-end collision is described as 6 o'clock. Three o'clock describes the collision into the passenger door, and the driver's door will be at 9 o'clock.

Newton's laws of motion

Newton's first law of motion is that an object in motion will remain in motion at the same speed and in the same direction until acted upon by an outside force. Newton's second law is that force is the product of mass and acceleration (F=ma); an object being pushed harder than another object of the same mass will move faster, and an object heavier than another object will move slower with the same force used on both objects. Newton's third law of motion is that for every action, there is an equal and opposite reaction. All three laws of motion can be applied to motor vehicle collisions. For instance, if applying Newton's second law of motion to a motor vehicle collision, two stationary vehicles hit from the rear by a third vehicle will move at different acceleration rates based upon size. A semi-truck will accelerate slower than a Ford Focus because of its size.

To utilize Newton's laws of motion, it is helpful to remember that the occupant will likely move toward the direction of impact. Thus, in a frontal collision, the occupant in the vehicle will be forced toward the front of the vehicle. In a read-end collision, the occupant will be forced toward the rear of the automobile. Side collisions will move the occupant toward the side of the vehicle hit. In a passenger side collision, the occupant will move toward the passenger side, and in a driver's side collision, the passenger will be forced toward the driver's side of the vehicle. The LNC will not be responsible for determining the load on the passengers in a vehicle, but should be aware of the impact implications. The load will be determined by the accident reconstructionist. This determination is based upon the change in velocity, with a greater load resulting in greater chance of injury.

Copyright © Mometrix Media. You have been licensed one copy of this document for personal use only. Any other reproduction or redistribution is strictly prohibited. All rights reserved.

Motor vehicle collision

Factors affecting severity of injuries

The factors involved might include a frontal collision versus a side collision and the speed of each vehicle just before the vehicles collide. The velocities of each vehicle, including changes in velocity, will impact the collision. Also, the sizes and masses of each vehicle will be a determining factor, as will the location and body position of each occupant. Safety equipment such as seat belts, and the proper use of each, can affect the severity of injuries. The parties' awareness of the accident can be a factor, since awareness can allow time to change position or restrain oneself. Also, the person's status, such as age, size, etc., can play a role in whether or not he/she suffers injuries.

Different types of motor vehicle collisions

The frontal, rear-end, side, and rollover are the main types of motor vehicle collisions. The LNC should, therefore, review the collision as it relates to the injuries sustained by the claimant. The type of collision will affect the type of injuries sustained by the vehicle's occupant(s). Generally, an injury is determined by the direction of force and the location of the individual in the vehicle. Both of these factors result in a general pattern. Further, the general pattern of injuries can usually disclose whether the vehicle's occupant was wearing a seat belt at the time of impact. The LNC must also be aware that a vehicle's occupant may suffer impact from several directions dependent upon the sequence of events involved in the collision (e.g., if a vehicle is hit from behind, causing it to be pushed into the vehicle in front).

Frontal collision in a motor vehicle accident

The frontal collision involves force exerted upon the vehicle's front end, between the 10 o'clock and 2 o'clock positions. The majority are offset frontal collisions (somewhere between 10 and 11 o'clock or between 1 and 2 o'clock), rather than head-on. The results experienced in offset collisions are different from head-on impacts. Offset collisions may experience force in less area than a head-on collision that will impact the entire front. The vehicle's occupant will travel toward the front of the automobile. The vehicle will likely stop, but the occupant will not because he/she is not a fixed part of the vehicle. This type of collision can also cause damage to the "survival zone" of the vehicle's passenger compartment, resulting in the engine block forced into the compartment. In this type, airbags are meant to deploy. The airbag, however, should deploy only at a certain speed,

Copyright © Mometrix Media. You have been licensed one copy of this document for personal use only. Any other reproduction or redistribution is strictly prohibited. All rights reserved.

usually 10 miles per hour. A head-on collision is also a frontal collision. A head-on collision can result in a vehicle hitting an object, such as a pole, or another vehicle.

Rear-end collision in a motor vehicle accident

Obviously, a rear-end collision involves a vehicle hit in the rear, either as a result of another vehicle hitting it or backing into an object. A rear-end collision can happen when a vehicle is at a stop and hit from behind by a moving vehicle. In this instance, the vehicle will be pushed forward and the occupant will remain in his/her position until struck by the back of the seat and/or head restraint. The occupant will be forced back into the padding of the seat, at which point his/her motion will slow down. This movement is known as the ride-down. A greater force can cause the neck to hyperextend (bend backward) and then hyperflex (bend forward). As a result, neck injuries are the most commonly alleged injuries in rear-end collisions. The impact from behind can also cause the seat back to break. Also, in older pick-up trucks, the head may strike the rear window because of lack of head restraint.

Side (lateral) collision in a motor vehicle accident

The side collision can occur in two ways. The first is the sideswipe. In this instance, the two vehicle involved in the collision are nearly parallel at the time of impact. The side collision is the second type of lateral collision. In this instance, one vehicle is hit on the side by the front end of another vehicle (forming a 'T' shape and known as a T-bone collision). This type of collision occurs most often at intersections. A collision on the side and at the location of the occupant of a vehicle is likely to cause injury, since there is limited space between the vehicles at the point of impact. Injuries occurring on the same side as impact may also result from objects protruding into the passenger compartment (e.g., a tree entering the vehicle on the impact side). In an impact occurring on the opposite side of the occupant's location in the vehicle, a loose object moving through the vehicle can cause injury. A common injury sustained in a side collision is a head injury.

Rollover collision in a motor vehicle accident

The types of rollover collisions include a collision followed by a rollover and a simple rollover involving no collision. Two dangers of this type of collision are ejection and the head impacting the ceiling. In fact, a rollover accident is the most common reason for ejection from a vehicle, especially if seat belts are not utilized. Another consideration will be the extent of crush to the roof. Generally, injuries sustained from rollover accidents tend

Copyright © Mometrix Media. You have been licensed one copy of this document for personal use only.
Any other reproduction or redistribution is strictly prohibited. All rights reserved.

to be either very serious (e.g., death or paralysis) or minor. There appears to be no in-between relative to injuries. As far as vehicle safety, sport utility vehicles may be subject to rollover incidents when execute certain maneuvers (e.g., sudden turns).

Three separate collisions sustained in one motor vehicle collision

Three separate collisions occur when a motor vehicle collision happens. In a front-end collision, the vehicle hits an object (the first collision), the vehicle's occupant then moves forward and is stopped by a vehicle restraint (the second collision), and then the occupant's internal structures are subject to the forces of the impact (the third collision). Injuries sustained a as a result of the various impacts include internal organ injury; bone fractures; muscle, tendon, ligament, or joint injury; head injury; scarring; neck and back injury; or soft tissue injury. In addition, an occupant may suffer deceleration injuries, which can cause tears in internal structures. Thermal and respiratory tract injuries can result from fire or explosion. Drowning may result if a vehicle comes to rest in water deep enough to submerge the vehicle. A smaller vehicle may be subject to having the top taken off by a larger vehicle (e.g., sedan collision with a semi-truck).

Seat belts

Seat belts can be essential in preventing injuries, especially ejection from the vehicle. The seat belt normally is the three-point type, although some vehicles have only a lap belt in the rear seats. In some instances, the seat belt latch has been reported to fail. In this instance, the occupant may have failed to properly latch the belt. However, some literature indicates some forces can cause the seat belt to unlatch. Also, occupants sometimes fail to wear seat belts in an appropriate fashion. For instance, the occupant may fail to latch the lap belt in a vehicle with a passive shoulder harness. This failure can contribute to the occupant's injuries, since the seat belt will be less efficient. Last, the seat belt can cause injuries, known as the "seat belt syndrome." The bruising resulting from a seat belt is known as the "seat belt sign." The seat belt itself can cause internal injuries.

Airbags

The airbag has been required at the driver and passenger side of vehicles since 1999. The airbag is designed to slow the occupant's movement in a frontal collision and to keep the occupant's head, face, and chest from striking the steering wheel, windshield, or steering wheel. The airbag may not deploy in a collision that is not frontal, the speed did not meet a certain force, it is defective, or it is turned off. Injuries that may result from the airbag itself

- 41 -

Copyright © Mometrix Media. You have been licensed one copy of this document for personal use only.
Any other reproduction or redistribution is strictly prohibited. All rights reserved.

include, chemical burns (as much as second-degree); alkali keratitis; eye injuries; hearing loss; hand, cervical vertebrae, and rib fractures; maxillofacial fractures; or diaphragmatic rupture. A small occupant, such as a child, or an individual sitting too close to the airbag area can more readily suffer injuries. Injuries sustained as a result of sitting too close to the airbag can result from the airbag module cover.

Restraints

First, the head restraint can aid in supporting the head in the event of a rear-end collision. The head restraint may prevent hyperextension, but must be adjusted properly based upon the occupant's height. Second, the infant car seat is required by states for infants. The vehicle's driver/owner should be certain that the infant car seat is properly installed and that the proper seat is utilized. Any seat other than an approved infant car seat is not appropriate for safe use in the vehicle. Third, child booster seats are designed to reduce or prevent injuries in a collision. Not all states require the use of child booster seats, but many are starting to do so. The child booster seat is normally recommended for a child who is not required to be in an infant car seat. The seat is designed to raise the child to allow a proper fit of the lap and shoulder belt.

Definitions

- Bullet vehicle: The bullet vehicle is the vehicle that runs into another vehicle.
- Target vehicle: The target vehicle is the vehicle that gets struck, either by a bullet vehicle or another object.
- A-pillar: The A-pillar is a support pillar for the passenger compartment located at the front corner of a vehicle.
- B-pillar: The B-pillar is a support pillar for the passenger compartment located between the front seat and back seat of a vehicle.
- Delta v: The delta v refers to the change in velocity of a vehicle as a result of a collision impact.
- Gs: The Gs refer to the unit of measurement for the acceleration or deceleration of a vehicle and is used to describe the load on an occupant as a result of a collision. A person or thing on the surface of the earth experiences one G (the force of gravity).

Copyright © Mometrix Media. You have been licensed one copy of this document for personal use only. Any other reproduction or redistribution is strictly prohibited. All rights reserved.

Pedestrian accident

Pedestrians are, of course, more likely to suffer severe injury in the case of a collision with a motor vehicle because they do not have impact protection. In fact, in this type of accident, a high risk of fatality exists since the pedestrian sustains the entire impact. The injuries sustained will be dependent upon several factors, including speed of the vehicle, physical attributes of the pedestrian, and the make-up of the vehicle's front end. Injuries may be sustained when a pedestrian lands on the hood of the vehicle, then impacts the ground. Also, being pulled under the vehicle's tires is a possible action. Sometimes, adults will be struck in the lower extremity, being knocked to the ground upon impact. As a result of ground impact, adults frequently suffer fractures, thoracic and abdominal injuries, and upper-extremity and craniofacial injuries. On the other hand, children tend to suffer crush injuries. Their size, much smaller than an adult, puts them at risk of being run over.

Medical records

The individuals who respond to the scene and those that transport the victim note facts that may be pertinent to the claimant's condition immediately, or shortly, after an accident. The records may contain information such as the vehicle exit route of the victim (door, window, etc.), a drawing of the location/type of injuries, including objective signs; claimant's consciousness or lack thereof; and whether the victim made any statements. Also, the data might indicate claimant's activity level (standing, sitting, etc.) and behavior at the scene. The victim's complaints, as well as vital signs and treatment provided should be contained in the record. What form of immobilization was used during transport, if any, should be noted. Last, the damage to the vehicle may be detailed, as well as any indication of use of restrain devices by the victim.

Documents

The written record of a motor vehicle collision involves a number of documents in addition to the medical records of the parties involved. The records can be utilized by the LNC to gather additional information or confirmation of a claimant's injuries, such as the type of injury sustained in relation to the type of collision. The traffic accident report, or police report, will be prepared by the law enforcement officer at the scene and will contain information such as collision details and statements taken. The law enforcement personnel at the scene may also taken photographs that the LNC can review to confirm the angle of vehicles or damage sustained. An estimate of vehicle repairs will also detail the damage to the vehicle. If the insurance adjuster records a statement of any party to the collision, this

Copyright © Mometrix Media. You have been licensed one copy of this document for personal use only.
Any other reproduction or redistribution is strictly prohibited. All rights reserved.

may be available for review. Last, the insurance adjuster or an attorney involved with the claim may retain an accident reconstructionist. If so, the LNC should obtain a copy of the report, although the LNC should review the report keeping in mind the party for whom it was prepared.

Accident report

The report will list the date, time, and location, as well as the drivers' information (e.g., name, address, etc.). The report may also describe the scene, including a drawing, and information regarding each vehicle involved. The damages to the vehicles may be listed, as well as the location of damage to each, and whether any vehicle involved had obvious mechanical defects. Collision information may include the type of collision, contributing factors, seating positions of occupants, restraint use for adults and children, and safety systems (e.g., airbag and deployment, bicycle helmet use). Other contributing factors might be alcohol or drug influence, roadway conditions, weather, lighting, pedestrian information (if applicable). The parties' insurance information will be on the form, as will statements of drivers and witnesses, if possible. Scene measurements will be noted, including location of physical evidence. The law enforcement officer will include his/her judgment of the accident's cause and responsibility and the tickets issued, including vehicle code sections violated. The report may also note whether photographs were taken, the parties' injury complaints, and transport information for each injured party.

Potential defendants

Review of the accident report and additional records will help the LNC and attorney determine the appropriate parties to name as defendants in a claim. Obviously, the driver of the vehicle impacting plaintiff or plaintiff's vehicle will be a named defendant. In addition, the plaintiff may name the owner of the vehicle (which may be a different individual than the driver). If the defendant was operating the vehicle during the course of employment, his/her employer may be named as a defendant. In the case of vehicle defects, the manufacturer of the vehicle or the manufacturer of a part or component may be designated a defendant. If the vehicle defect was caused by a negligent repair, the pertinent individuals of the repair facility will be defendants. The entity or municipality responsible for the roadway can be a defendant, if plaintiff's attorney find lack of proper design or maintenance to be a factor in the collision.

Copyright © Mometrix Media. You have been licensed one copy of this document for personal use only.
Any other reproduction or redistribution is strictly prohibited. All rights reserved.

Premises liability

- Slip and fall: If a person's foot slips on a flooring surface, a fall may occur. Two types may occur: backward falls result from slipping of the forward foot or a fall occurs because the rear foot slips backward. A foreign substance can also cause a foot to slip.

- Trip and fall: Normally, this fall happens because a person's foot impacts or catches an object or projection. The foot stops, but the upper body continues forward.

- Step and fall: When a step forward results in an unexpected step down, a forward fall occurs.

- Fall due to loss of consciousness and other conditions: A loss of consciousness can result in a fall. This fall can cause injury to the face, since there is usually no attempt to stop the impact. Also, an individual may lose his/her balance or experience vertigo.

- Failure of lower extremity: Failure of any lower extremity can cause an individual to fall. This type of failure may result from osteoporosis or bone metastasis conditions, a twisted ankle, knee problems, or hip issues.

Falls from a height and falls on or down stairs

- Falls from a height: This type of fall usually involve ladders, step stools, trees, windows, roofs, or beds. The injury sustained may be dictated by the height of the fall; obviously, a greater distance normally results in more severe injuries. Also, the landing surface and position on impact will determine injuries. The party may suffer back injuries if he/she lands on his/her feet (e.g., compression fracture in lumbar spine area). Additionally, head injuries abdominal injuries, thoracic visceral injuries, and wrist injuries may result.

- Falls on or down stairs: Injuries sustained from this fall may be severe as a result of the height of the stairs, the momentum as the party falls, and the probable tumbling motion of the body. An expert will investigate the height of the stair, friction issues, and slope.

Preparing review of a personal injury case

The LNC will normally receive a telephone call from an attorney to review a possible injury claim. Upon acceptance of the assignment, the LNC will request copies of the medical

- 45 -

Copyright © Mometrix Media. You have been licensed one copy of this document for personal use only. Any other reproduction or redistribution is strictly prohibited. All rights reserved.

records, as well as additional reports and records that may have been prepared. The LNC must then organize the records for review. After organization, the LNC will review the records and prepare a summary of the collision and injuries sustained. The LNC will also prepare a chronological record of the incident and plaintiff's care. If the LNC notes any missing records, those must be requested to complete the report. Once the complete set of records have been obtained and reviewed, the LNC will prepare a detailed summary for the attorney's review. Thereafter, it might be necessary for the LNC to obtain medical literature. At this point, the LNC should have all pertinent information to analyze the accident and injuries sustained. After analysis, the LNC will meet with the attorney to provide and discuss the report.

Strict liability action

To maintain a strict liability claim, the plaintiff must prove the product was sold by the manufacturer, it was defective, there is a causal relationship between the defect and injuries, and the plaintiff has been damaged. With strict liability, the plaintiff does not have to show fault. This liability centers on the product and its safety. The LNC should keep in mind that drugs and medical devices require a different perspective, since these products are generally subject to some side effects. In addition, the LNC should be aware that under the Restatement (Second) of Torts, Sec. 402A, Comment k, some drugs have been deemed unsafe, but the benefits justify the risks. Under this circumstance, the manufacturer must provide a sufficient warning to utilize this defense.

National Vaccine Injury Act

The National Vaccine Injury Act was created in 1986 by Congress, and any claim for injuries resulting from vaccines must now be applied under the Act. This Act created a "no-fault" compensation program for vaccine manufacturers granting liability protection. This protection alleviates concern regarding loss due to claims. Children suffering vaccine hypersensitivity reactions can also acquire compensation without court action. Under an amendment in 1995, a claimant must now show he/she suffered symptoms and they were not present before the vaccination. If a claimant cannot show causation, he/she must demonstrate appearance of symptoms within three days of vaccination. Finally, in 1997, an amendment provided that future vaccines are included in this Act.

Copyright © Mometrix Media. You have been licensed one copy of this document for personal use only. Any other reproduction or redistribution is strictly prohibited. All rights reserved.

Product liability negligence claim

Negligence is demonstrated when conduct is less than the accepted standard designed to protect individuals from unreasonable damages or injuries. Essential to a negligence claim is the defendant's conduct. The plaintiff must demonstrate a duty, breach of duty, damages, and proximate cause. For example, if a drug manufacturer fails to recall a drug even after unexplained injuries occur, the company may be subject to negligence. In this instance, FDA approval could not be used as a defense.

Definitions

- Defective design: This theory refers to a drug or device deemed unsafe for the purpose intended or a purpose that can be expected. This theory may apply when the drug or device is made to specifications, but is then inadequate or subject to substantial side effects. This includes all products made to the same specifications.
- Defective manufacture: This theory applies when a product is defective due to its manufacturing process, and is defective at the time it leaves the manufacturer's control.
- Failure to warn: This theory is effective when a product label fails to provide adequate warnings regarding the use of the product (normally drug or device actions). If a relationship between injury and a drug or device occurs after labeling, the FDA requires the manufacturer to revise the label, augment the insert, or notify physicians.
- Learned intermediary: In the area of product liability actions, the learned intermediary is the individual or entity responsible for transfer of information provided by a manufacturer to the person receiving the product from the intermediary. For instance, a physician is responsible for providing information to a patient when prescribing drugs or medical devices, rather than the manufacturer. The patient, therefore, relies upon the physician and not the manufacturer. Learned intermediary provides protection to manufacturers, unless the label information is ultimately insufficient.
- Over-the-counter products: Over-the-counter products include FDA Class II devices available without prescription. In this instance, the product labeling must be sufficient to advise the consumer of possible hazards. The labeling must be understandable by a layperson.

Copyright © Mometrix Media. You have been licensed one copy of this document for personal use only. Any other reproduction or redistribution is strictly prohibited. All rights reserved.

Manufacturers criteria

- Knowledge of the risk: The manufacturer must be aware of the possible adverse effects of the product at the time it became available to consumers. The manufacturer is considered an expert relative to the product distributed.
- The nature and timing of the duty to warn: The manufacturer must warn the consumer of risks not only at the time of distribution, but continually throughout the life of the product on the market.
- Language used to convey the warning: Labeling to convey a warning must be on the product, as well as supplement the product. All writings and verbal communications regarding the product constitute labeling.

Proper drug product labeling

The Food and Drug Administration controls the format and content of labels on drug products. Warnings, contraindications, indications, precautions, and dosage are among the information to be placed on the label. This regulation applies to supplemental labeling. The FDA must approve the proposed label as part of the approval process. The information must be stated in such a fashion to meet federal guidelines. The FDA can determine a label is insufficient if the facts contained on it are lacking, the response is unreasonably delayed, or the language used is not strong enough. In other words, the language must conform with the risk involved. Warnings must be highly visible, as well as clear and understandable.

Food and Drug Administration

The Food, Drug, and Cosmetic Act of 1938 was the parent act of the current Food and Drug Administration. The 1938 Act was designed to increase the government's regulation of drugs, including the requirement that new drugs be proved safe prior to consumer marketing. As a result of the 1938 Act, which initiated prescriptions for many drugs, the FDA was established. Thereafter, it became the responsibility of the FDA to monitor the marketing for new drugs. The Kefauver-Harris Amendment of 1962 was then enacted to strictly monitor the safety and labeling of drugs; this Amendment was established as a

- 48 -

Copyright © Mometrix Media. You have been licensed one copy of this document for personal use only. Any other reproduction or redistribution is strictly prohibited. All rights reserved.

result of thalidomide's adverse side effects. The FDA now concentrates on locating adverse reactions and conveying information to the public.

New drugs

All United States medical and pharmaceutical products are under the administration of the FDA. The FDA's procedure is designed to lessen the possibility that consumers will be subjected to risks from new drugs. Thus, before the FDA can approve release to consumers, a drug must be tested for safety and effectiveness. To meet FDA approval, the manufacturer must subject the drug to clinical trials. Although a major consideration in the safety of new drugs, the clinical trial tests only a small portion of the public. The trials contrast results from two or more groups, with one receiving the drug and one receiving a placebo or other therapy.

Three phases of testing prior to submitting a new drug application
The manufacturer must perform three phases of testing before submitting a new drug application to the FDA. The testing is designed to show safety and effectiveness for the drug.
- Phase 1 trials involve determining the highest dose subjects can endure. Normally, the individuals involved in this phase are healthy. The target market is addressed in
- Phase 2, when the drug's effectiveness and safety are tested on a small model of this segment.
- In Phase 3, random, blind, and placebo-controlled studies are performed. In this instance, neither the researcher or the subjects are aware of actual drug versus placebo submission. All three phases of testing are monitored by the FDA.

FDA procedure after clinical trials
The FDA will grant the new drug application if the research and testing have been completed and results are satisfactory. The Prescription Drug User Fee Act of 1992 allows manufacturers to pay a fee to speed the process for approval of the new drug application. As a result, in 1997, new drugs were approved within an average of 10.8 months. The FDA is attempting to make the process time even less lengthy. Based upon the new drug application's approval, consumers should be able to expect a drug is safe if used properly (e.g., approved indication, proper dose, a limited time of use). Of course, the clinical trials

Copyright © Mometrix Media. You have been licensed one copy of this document for personal use only.
Any other reproduction or redistribution is strictly prohibited. All rights reserved.

utilized to obtain approval involve a limited number of individuals. Thus, not all side effects can be determined appropriately until the drug has been used by a larger population for an extended period of time.

Monitoring post-marketing of drugs

Currently, the FDA does not have the prerogative to order manufacturers to conduct post-marketing clinical trials. If trials do occur after marketing, they are done willingly by the manufacturer. Manufacturers find it too time costly and financially expensive to delay offering a drug to consumers until they are able to determine all possible risks. Also, manufacturers feel it is unethical to withhold a drug they deem effective. However, manufacturers need to continue observing drugs after marketing to determine issues that may arise. Also, monitoring drugs after marketing assists in determining reactions in populations other than those used in trials, as well as ascertaining effects that may occur after a lengthy period.

Informed consent in clinical trials

Human subjects were used in clinical trials without their consent mostly during World War II. Those studies resulted in abuses to the subjects in the trials. As a result, several key rules have been adopted to regulate clinical trials. The Nuremberg Code of 1949 sets forth the rules for such experiments and required voluntary consent of individuals. The Declaration of Helsinki of 1964 is designed to assist physicians and medical personnel to maintain ethical principles when using human beings in medical research. The Belmont Report of 1979 encompasses the ethical principles and guidelines involved in human research. The Good Clinical Practice Guidelines (GCP) set forth the standards for all areas of trials. The trial subject must voluntarily sign and date a consent for research, which must also be witnessed and approved by the Institutional Review Board. The subject must sign the form prior to the trial's commencement. The subject must also be aware of risks and understand the research.

Serious adverse event occurrences (SAEs)

The entity investigating the proposed drug must report all SAEs immediately when known. This report shall be made to the sponsor group (usually the manufacturer). The sponsor

Copyright © Mometrix Media. You have been licensed one copy of this document for personal use only. Any other reproduction or redistribution is strictly prohibited. All rights reserved.

must then advise the Food and Drug Administration and investigators. The notification must take place through a written IND safety report. 21 CRF Sec. 312.32 defines an SAE as death, life-threatening reactions, reactions that lengthen or require hospitalization, congenital anomalies or birth defects, prolonged or serious disability or incapacity, or an occurrence that might compromise the patient in any of the above manners.

LNC's review

When reviewing medical records, the LNC should first determine whether the claimant was part of a clinical trial. If the LNC determines this is relevant from the records, the LNC should first locate the consent form. The consent form would then be reviewed by the LNC to determine that it meets all specifications and approval by the Institutional Review Board and other applicable agencies. The LNC should obtain all records pertaining to the clinical trial for review. The documents requested would include the informed consent, Institutional Review Board paperwork, the study protocol, and study patient source documents. The LNC can then review the records to determine that proper protocol was followed and the claimant was, in fact, eligible to act as a subject in the trial.

1976 Medical Device Amendment of the Food, Drug, and Cosmetic Act

The Medical Device Amendment allowed the Food and Drug Administration to monitor medical devices. Prior to enactment, medical devices were not subject to review prior to marketing. As a result of the amendment, medical devices are now subject to regulation much like that used for drugs. The term "medical device" covers any item manufactured or marketed for a medical purpose without reliance on chemical action. The approval of medical devices is not based upon safety and effectiveness like drugs; it is based upon risk. Approval is based upon whether the device meets safety and effectiveness guidelines in light of its intended use. The manufacturer does not have to prove that using the device is without risk.

Regulatory classes for medical devices
- Class I: These devices must meet good manufacturing practices to be marketable.
- Class II: These devices are not subject to premarketing approval (PMA). They are, however, subject to quality control requirements during manufacturing.

Copyright © Mometrix Media. You have been licensed one copy of this document for personal use only. Any other reproduction or redistribution is strictly prohibited. All rights reserved.

- Class III: These devices are subject to the premarketing approval (PMA) process. Devices that are considered essential, will be implanted, or when failure will threaten the life of the consumers are in this class.

As a general rule, medical devices are not controlled by Food and Drug Administration as closely as drugs.

FDA's spontaneous reporting system

Manufacturers must monitor drugs after marketed to the public. If complications occur, these must be reported to the FDA. Complications are defined as an adverse effect that is connected to the drug, even if it is not specifically drug-related. The report by the manufacturer must be submitted to the FDA within 15 days of knowledge of a serious occurrence. The FDA may request the drug be removed from the market, or the manufacturer may do so by choice. The FDA may learn of negative effects through the reports filed by physicians to manufacturers or directly to the FDA. However, the health care provider must notify the FDA directly if a death or hospitalization results from a vaccine. A party involved in a product liability action may utilize an adverse drug reaction report as evidence.

Downside of the FDA's spontaneous reporting system

The system does not insure the safety of a drug. It does, however, grant the public early notice of possible health risks. The reports made by physicians and manufacturers notifying the FDA of adverse drug reactions may contain many opinions, rather than facts. The reports may also provide too much unnecessary information. Results may be misinterpreted by the reporting party. The risks may be under-reported by physicians and manufacturers; in fact, this is a serious issue. The physician may provide an impartial opinion in his/her report or the information may be so cumbersome that it affects the system. Based upon the negative issues involved with the spontaneous reporting system, actual rates of adverse reactions cannot be determined from the information.

FDA's MEDWatch system

The Medical Products Reporting Program (MEDWatch) was developed by the Food and Drug Administration in June 1993. This program is designed to guarantee health care

Copyright © Mometrix Media. You have been licensed one copy of this document for personal use only. Any other reproduction or redistribution is strictly prohibited. All rights reserved.

providers will not only identify, but also report adverse drug and medical device effects. As a result of this requirement, the FDA and manufacturers are made aware of risks, and safety issues can be properly addressed. Because clinical trials are limited, manufacturers and the FDA must be aware of interactions that were not available during pre-marketing studies. The program provides a simple process for health care providers to report to the FDA. The program also provides the FDA with information about medical device risks, product label issues, packaging issues, contamination, or instability of drugs or devices.

Product liability actions

Case analysis of drug/medical device
First, the LNC should determine that the health care provider exercised the proper standard of care when the drug or medical device was prescribed. Second, the LNC should review all records relative to the claimant, including medical, military, employment, education, and criminal. Third, in the case of defense strategy, the LNC should determine whether an action should be brought against a third party. Fourth, the LNC must show a causal relationship between the drug/medical device and the claimant's injuries. Fifth, the LNC must research the drug/medical device. Sixth, the LNC should obtain the medical device reports and adverse drug reactions reports from the FDA, which are available to the public. Seventh, the LNC should compile or obtain epidemiological evidence. Eighth, the LNC must review all records and data compiled. Last, the LNC should enlist medical and technical experts to be used as witnesses as trial.

Ruling out medical negligence
Ruling out medical negligence is the main responsibility of the LNC when reviewing a product liability action. The LNC should review the standard of care relative to the health care provider prescribing the drug or medical device. Obviously, the manufacturer may not be held liable if the health care provider failed to prescribe the drug or medical device in accordance with recommendations. In this instance, the health care provider may be solely liable for the injuries sustained. In addition, the medical records of the claimant should be reviewed regarding possible misdiagnosis, below-standard medical treatment, or insufficient follow-up treatment by any practitioner.

Copyright © Mometrix Media. You have been licensed one copy of this document for personal use only. Any other reproduction or redistribution is strictly prohibited. All rights reserved.

Plaintiff's medical history

The medical, mental health, employment, education, criminal, and military records of the claimant should be completely reviewed when establishing a product liability claim. The records should be reviewed with the knowledge that a drug-induced illness might be hard to identify with a patient suffering from several contemporaneous illnesses. Also, the LNC must completely review the claimant's pharmaceutical history, since it will help determine drug-drug interactions, contraindications relative to the drug use being reviewed, whether the drug (including a similar drug) was previously taken with no complications, or overuse of the drug. Alcohol should also be reviewed as a contributing factor relative to alleged injuries. The LNC should review all records with the applicable statute of limitations in mind, since the dates of prescriptions, product use, or device implantation/failure may impact the claim.

Establishing a causal relationship

The LNC will assist the attorney in establishing a causal relationship between the claimant's injury and the drug or device utilized. The drug or device utilized by the claimant must be the active cause between the use and resultant injury with no interference from another source. As an LNC on behalf of a claimant, he/she should review the records not only to determine the drug or device in question was the cause of the injury, but to omit any contributing factors. In causation, the "but for" rule may be applied, allowing that an initial event causes a second event when that event would not have happened but for the initial event. It may be hard to prove undeniably that the prescribed drug or device caused the alleged injuries.

LNC's research practice

The LNC will research medical literature relative to the product in question, both before litigation and during the lawsuit. The LNC must be aware of the claimant's use of the product, as well as the indications and their effect on the claimant's end result. The LNC should be aware that the drug or device label will be referred to regularly during the litigation process. Thus, the LNC should be familiar with the label in question, as well as all warnings during the claimant's time of use. The LNC should also be familiar with all advertisements published by the manufacturer and the effect upon the label and package insert. A cross-search of computer online services should be conducted relative to similar drugs or devices and like injuries as a result. Positive and negative information relative to the claim will be helpful to the attorney, so the LNC should not overlook negative

Copyright © Mometrix Media. You have been licensed one copy of this document for personal use only. Any other reproduction or redistribution is strictly prohibited. All rights reserved.

information. The dates of all pertinent information should be noted to establish the manufacturer's duty to keep abreast of knowledge regarding the product.

Obtaining adverse reaction and medical device reports

The LNC should request from the Food and Drug Administration all Medical Device Reports and Adverse Reaction Reports relative to the product alleged to have caused the injury. The Freedom of Information Act provides that all citizens are entitled to request and obtain this information from the FDA. The LNC can utilize the Act to request the records from the FDA. The LNC should be aware, also, that the response to a request to the FDA will take a long time. Also, the FDA will not provide information regarding drugs or devices that are still in the investigation phase and have not yet been approved. In this case, the LNC must utilize medical literature and computer databases to obtaining relevant information regarding the drug or device. When responding to the LNC's request, the FDA may provide a computerized tabulation of the reports. Important to the plaintiff's claim is the fact that the reports will not establish cause and effect to prove the claim.

Identifying epidemiological studies and evidence

As the LNC is aware, epidemiology is the study of disease in people. Epidemiologists are specialists in the field of disease as it relates to occurrence and distribution. The LNC should be aware that epidemiology studies related to the claim must meet certain criteria to negate bias and error. The epidemiologist will be able to provide information relative to the reliability of the studies and whether the studies can prove cause and effect. The epidemiologist will be concerned with studies that demonstrate statistically relevant evidence that the claimant is part of a group that has received exposure to a drug or toxin at the level and during the period necessary to result in a negative effect. The epidemiologist will be able to show the causal relationship between the claimed injuries and the scientific information. The role of the LNC will be to insure the experts retained have sufficient knowledge of the strength and weakness of the data relevant to the claim.

Obtaining medical experts

The LNC will assist in obtaining qualified technical and medical experts to testify regarding the medical issues and the issues regarding design and manufacture of a product, warning progression, epidemiological studies, and marketing. The experts should be able to explain this information in a manner understandable to the jury. The LNC should search for experts who have performed research or clinical trials or written articles relative to the

Copyright © Mometrix Media. You have been licensed one copy of this document for personal use only. Any other reproduction or redistribution is strictly prohibited. All rights reserved.

product. The LNC should also locate experts possessing awareness of the product, including known adverse reactions, metabolism, indications, and method of action. The expert(s) chosen should be familiar with literature to support the testimony and be able to show their knowledge and experience relative to the product. The trial judge will determine the admissibility of the expert's testimony and evidence prior to presentation to the jury. Therefore, the LNC must provide medical experts capable of supporting the plaintiff's theories of the action. The expert is retained mainly to educate the jury. The LNC should insure that the expert has reviewed all records before testifying, that he/she understands the issues of the action; and that he/she possesses a strong opinion regarding the issues.

Definitions
- Air pollution: This is a broad term that includes visible elements of pollution such as smoke, smog, and haze.
- Chemical substances: This is a general term for basic elements and complex chemical compounds.
- Carcinogenicity: The likelihood of a chemical to cause cancer as scientifically established.
- Chronic risks: These risks appear as a result of repeated contact with a chemical substance over a prolonged period.
- Sick-building syndrome: This term is used to illustrate a group of symptoms that may occur in office environments, especially in buildings that are sealed and controlled through central ventilation systems.
- Define citizen suits, environmental releases, latency period, and dose-response effect relative to toxic tort claims
- Citizen suits: This type of lawsuit is a statutory action designed to enforce penalty provisions of the federal environmental laws, but is brought by an individual rather than a federal agency.
- Environmental releases: These represent the liquids, solids, and gases that are released by a facility into the outside environment through sewage, landfills, etc.
- Latency period: The extended time period between the claimant's exposure to a toxin and the onset of illness.
- Dose-response effect: The effect on living organisms of an alleged toxic material; a chemical can be considered safe in small doses, but toxic in larger doses.

Copyright © Mometrix Media. You have been licensed one copy of this document for personal use only.
Any other reproduction or redistribution is strictly prohibited. All rights reserved.

Types of toxic tort cases
- Single-claimant case: This type of action involves a single claimant exposed to one or more chemicals in a single (acute) exposure or during a lengthy period chronic).
- Multilitigant case: This type of action involves several claimants who have experienced similar exposure. However, each claimant's medical claims may be different in type and severity. This type of litigation may result in the court with jurisdiction certifying a class action suit.
- Class action suit: This type of action involves many claimants acting as plaintiffs in litigation. The parties must meet the court's standards to certify the litigation as a class action. Normally, a representative, either an individual or an entity, is chosen to represent the plaintiffs.

Chemical exposure

The LNC must assist in determining the route of toxic exposure, whether inhaled or otherwise. Most toxic tort claims are a result of inhalation exposure, normally through the lungs. Inhalation can occur as a result of both gaseous chemicals (e.g., chlorine) and particulate matters (e.g., asbestos). This type of exposure can happen at work, home, or in the global environment. Inhalation exposures can cause respiratory-related illness, systemic and cardiovascular effects, or immune and nervous system alterations. Another form of exposure may be through ingestion. A claimant may accidentally swallow toxic substances at home or work. Also, the claimant may have ingested unwashed fruits or vegetables tainted with fertilizers or pesticides. Quantifying this type of exposure may be problematic. Direct skin contact with a toxic substance can result in cutaneous exposure. The skin does have a protective function, which can limit this type of exposure to localized reaction (e.g., rash, pruritus).

Labeling guidelines

The LNC will review in detail the labeling procedure and information relative to the product in question. The label must be accurate and contain storage information. Also, the label must state protective equipment and clothing that should be used when handling the substance, as well as appropriate disposal procedures. The Safety Data Sheet (SDS) will outline a compound's contents, health and fire hazards, appropriate first aid, and the ideal methods of use, storage, and disposal. The LNC should review the SDS forms for the time

Copyright © Mometrix Media. You have been licensed one copy of this document for personal use only. Any other reproduction or redistribution is strictly prohibited. All rights reserved.

period in question, as well as all changes made during a specified time period prior to and after the exposure. The Occupational Safety and Health Administration (OSHA) sets permissible exposure limits for approximately 500 hazardous chemicals. The American Conference of Governmental Industrial Hygienists (ACGIH) also sets permissible exposure limits through its Threshold Limit Value Committee and Ventilation Committee. These limits are utilized worldwide and, in some instances, are lower than OSHA's limits.

Causation

In a toxic tort case, causation requires establishing a connection between the exposure and the alleged injury. Normally, the "preponderance of the evidence" falls upon the plaintiff. In other words, the plaintiff must show that the injury resulted from the exposure. Demonstrating causation is not a simple matter in toxic tort claims, since the plaintiff must prove scientific causation. In order to prove this, statistical methods are utilized to show a high-confidence or statistically significant connection between the claimant's illness and his/her exposure. Not only must the injury be shown by the medical and social records, but the alleged toxic substance must be shown to cause the alleged injury. The latency period makes it difficult to prove the injury. This period allows time for the defendant to allege exposure to multiple harmful substances. Also, with low-level toxic substance exposure, the scientific proof may prove limited.

Defense tactics/allegations

The defense LNC will determine claimed injuries, attempting to disprove plaintiff's causation claim. The defense may attempt to visit the exposure site, which may fall to the LNC. Should a site visit be impossible, the LNC should review all information provided during discovery, searching specifically for the (lack of) presence of the product at the alleged exposure site. Obviously, this is done to prove the defendant's product cannot be found responsible. If the product can be traced to the site, the defense will attempt to allege the product was not stored or maintained properly, was not in an area that would cause plaintiff's exposure, or was not used properly. The LNC may try to prove the product did not cause the alleged injuries, or the injuries do not comply with those known to be caused by the substance. The LNC may also show that plaintiff contributed to his/her injury by failure to obtain timely treatment, by improper use of the product, or by failing to utilize safety equipment.

Copyright © Mometrix Media. You have been licensed one copy of this document for personal use only. Any other reproduction or redistribution is strictly prohibited. All rights reserved.

Social and employment records

The LNC should be aware that detailed information regarding the claimant is vital to showing a valid injury. Thus, both social and medical records combined will assist in this showing. The claimant's social records, from childhood to the date of review, can assist in determining congenital problems, traumatic events, debilitating childhood illnesses. Also, personal records may disclose a limited earning capability shown by neurological or IQ testing results. The occupational records may disclose information regarding additional sources of exposure or other risk factors. Employment records may reveal pre-employment physical examinations, laboratory test results, medical screenings, or attendance records. Under "right-to-know" legislation, these records may help confirm all places of employment complied with state and federal protection laws. The LNC should be mindful of plaintiff's habits, since everyday events can cause exposures of which claimant is unaware.

Failure to disclose medical information

The claimant may fail to disclose all medical information simply because of embarrassment. Plastic surgery, treatment for STDs, or psychiatric treatment may fall cause embarrassment. A claimant may also forget medical information if treatment occurred once or many years previous. The LNC can determine additional medical information to be obtained through review of the billings and medical records that reference previous treatments or names of other health care providers. The claimant may also attempt to falsify his/her current physical and mental conditions. Since the neurological and central nervous system injuries that result in toxic tort cases can be biased or imprecise, making measurement difficult, the LNC should consult expert neuropsychiatrists, neurologists, or other experts skilled in cognitive function. These experts can assist the LNC in making accurate determinations of injuries.

Evaluating a corporate defendant's history

A corporate defendant is required to provide all information requested during discovery. This information will include corporate activities and practices, which will involve the relationship between practices and alleged damages. The LNC may review the "in-house working papers" and documentation compiled and prepared during research, development, manufacturing, and marketing for the subject product. The in vivo and in vitro studies of cellular, animal, and human systems will probably be part of the documentation. The LNC should consider this documentation to be confidential and treat it

Copyright © Mometrix Media. You have been licensed one copy of this document for personal use only.
Any other reproduction or redistribution is strictly prohibited. All rights reserved.

as such during the course of litigation. The LNC may review the product's material data safety sheet inserts and package labeling. The LNC should keep in mind that the claim against the corporate defendant may be difficult to prove.

Experts in a toxic tort case and their field of practice

The experts involved in toxic tort cases may include toxicologists, epidemiologists, safety engineers, industrial hygienists, and physicians. The toxicologist can evaluate toxic substances and effects upon living organisms. This expert may be able to explain or rebut the methods employed for evaluation or testing regarding the substance. The causal link between the disease and the existence in the population at large may be determined by the epidemiologist. Physicians retained as experts may include neuropsychologists or neuropsychiatrists to testify regarding cognitive function and changes, as well as those experts in occupational medicine, immunology, pulmonology, or oncology.

Reviewing literature

The LNC may be called upon to provide factual data supporting plaintiff's claim or defendant's position. The literature should provide illnesses and known symptoms associated with the product in question, including specific information regarding acute and chronic exposures for both human beings and animals. The literature should encompass the time frame in question, as well as current information. The search may disclose documentation published in foreign journals. The LNC should not discard this literature, but should search for English abstracts to determine the value of the article or retain a translator. The translator must be certified to provide authenticity in the translation. The LNC should be aware of the Daubert standards applied to medical evidence.

The Daubert standards and the Federal Rules of Evidence

These standards were established by Daubert vs. Merrell Dow Pharmaceuticals (1993). This case established the trial judge's role as gatekeeper in determining the admissibility of medical evidence. The trial judge will review the methodology, reliability, and relevance of testimony provided by experts. The judge will then determine whether the testimony is based upon valid scientific methodology and, thus, admissible as evidence. The Daubert standards are not used in all cases, but are being used more often. The Federal Rules of Evidence (FRE) do apply relative to expert witness testimony and evidence. The rules set forth the qualifications necessary for expert testimony, as well as the forms of data upon

Copyright © Mometrix Media. You have been licensed one copy of this document for personal use only. Any other reproduction or redistribution is strictly prohibited. All rights reserved.

which they may rely for opinions. FRE 401, 701, 702, and 703 encompass the rules that apply to experts.

Important terms

- TLV (Threshold limit value): This applies to the daily exposure an employee can sustain relative to airborne concentrations, measured in parts per million or billion (or milligrams per cubic meter in dermal exposure). The limit is 8 hours per day, 40 hours per week without harmful effects. This is also referred to as the time weighted average (TWA).
- PEL (Permissible exposure limit): This limit is comparable to the threshold limit value.
- STEL (Short-term exposure limit): This is a limited exposure in addition to the threshold limit value, which cannot surpass 15 minutes more than four times per day, and the employee must not sustain chronic tissue damage, irritation, or be unable to self-rescue. Also, each exposure must be at least 60 minutes apart.
- IDLH (Immediately dangerous to life and health): This provides the maximum concentration that an employee can sustain without suffering irreversible health effect or self-rescue impairment, with escape within 30 minutes.
- SDS (Safety data sheet): This form is required of manufacturers or vendors in all shipments of products containing chemical substances. The form sets forth the ingredients, the Chemical Abstracts Service registry identification, and information about exposure and handling.
- PPE (Personal protective equipment): This encompasses the clothing, masks and goggles, or respirators that must be worn to provide protection from exposure to chemicals and pathogens.

Copyright © Mometrix Media. You have been licensed one copy of this document for personal use only.
Any other reproduction or redistribution is strictly prohibited. All rights reserved.

Torts/Product Liability/Toxic Torts

Tort

Tort law represents civil law involving negligence, personal injury, and medical malpractice. The law is defined by three components: (1) a wrongful act must have occurred, (2) the act must cause injury to another person or property, and (3) judicial remedy must be possible. All three elements must be met to constitute a tort. Tort law is designed to grant an injured person corrective remedies through monetary compensation or damages. Further, the person(s) causing harm must have acted of his/her/their own free will, otherwise that person(s) cannot be held liable. The person(s) must also be able to understand the consequences of the act. For example, a intellectually disabled individual may be adjudged not liable.

Definitions

- Intentional Tort: A deliberate or intentional act violating or injuring another individual or the property of another individual. Intentional torts include assault and battery, trespass, or intentional infliction of emotional distress.
- Unintentional Tort: Also referred to as a "negligent tort." An unintentional act by one party against another that causes injury or harm. This form includes negligence and malpractice claims or an unintended automobile accident.
- Quasi-Intentional Tort: A tort that involves a form of speech, either oral or written. Basically, this tort is designed to protect individual privacy, reputation, or freedom from unfounded legal actions. Examples of this form of tort include slander and defamation.
- Toxic Tort: This form involves injury as a result of exposure to toxins (e.g., herbicides, pesticides, plutonium, radiation, emissions, or asbestos). This is a fairly recent form of tort law.
-

Four elements of negligence

- The health care provider must owe a duty of care to the patient. Normally, this duty arises upon the provider's acceptance of care and treatment responsibility of the patient.

Copyright © Mometrix Media. You have been licensed one copy of this document for personal use only. Any other reproduction or redistribution is strictly prohibited. All rights reserved.

- The health care provider must breach his/her duty or standard of care to the patient.
- The patient must show a proximate cause or causal connection between his/her damages or injuries suffered and the alleged breach of duty by the health care provider.
- The patient must suffer provable damages or injuries.

Define relevant, hearsay evidence, error-in-judgment rule, and two-schools-of-thought doctrine relative to standards of care

Relevant: Relevance, in general, pertains to evidence utilized to prove or disprove an issue. When utilized in standards of care, the evidence must be relevant to factual issues of the litigation. In this respect, the evidence must pertain not only to the subject, but the time in question.

Hearsay evidence: If a witness does not personally testify regarding the validity of evidence, the evidence may be considered hearsay evidence. Relative to standards of care, evidence may be considered hearsay if the author to a document pertaining to standards is not present as a witness.

Error-in-judgment rule: Relative to standards of care, this defense to malpractice provides that the health care provider met the standard of care despite the fact that an error occurred.

Two-schools-of-thought-doctrine: Relative to standards of care, this defense to malpractice provides that a health care provider is not negligent when one of several recognized, available treatment methods is adopted.

Four differences between negligence and intentional torts
- Intent: Unlike in a negligence action, the individual alleged to have perpetrated an intentional tort must have done so intending to interfere with the rights of another party, even if not done so in a hostile fashion.
- Proof of damages: Intentional torts hinder an individual's rights. In that event, the injured party does not have to prove an injury exists, since the damage is the

- 63 -

Copyright © Mometrix Media. You have been licensed one copy of this document for personal use only. Any other reproduction or redistribution is strictly prohibited. All rights reserved.

invasion of private right. In negligence actions, the injury represents the harm to the party.

- Duty or Standards of Care: Unintentional torts (negligence actions) require that duties or standards of care have been breached. Intentional torts do not involve duty or standards of care.
- Consent: A party's consent acts as an absolute defense when involved in intentional torts. In a negligence action, however, consent may not always act as a defense, as in the example of a patient consenting to surgery and then suffering injury as a result.

Measuring exposure in toxic tort cases

Before any litigation action is taken, the LNC and attorney must determine that exposure to a toxic substance has actually occurred. Therefore, this is an extremely important element in toxic tort actions. First, it must be confirmed that a toxic exposure has taken place. The exposure is measured by the "route" or means of exposure. This can include inhalation, oral ingestion, or cutaneous absorption. Second, the length of exposure must be ascertained. This length of exposure can be compared to safety guidelines set by regulatory agencies. Third, the frequency of the claimant's exposure must be determined. This may include periods ranging from a single (acute) exposure to that of extended (chronic) exposure. After making determinations of route, frequency, and duration, the LNC will collaborate with toxicologists or industrial hygienists to estimate the dose of exposure. The dose-response is determined to calculate the relationship between the level of exposure and increased risk of negative effects to the claimant.

Definitions
- Product liability: An area of law based on the premise that a manufacturer is responsible for the product placed on the market, and if defective, the manufacturer is subject to a lawsuit.
- Warranty: The manufacturer's promise that a product placed on the market is fit for the purpose sold. This includes quality, performance, and characteristics.
- Express warranty: A warranty about a product communicated to a consumer, either directly or indirectly.
- Implied warranty: A warranty occurring as a matter of law.

Copyright © Mometrix Media. You have been licensed one copy of this document for personal use only. Any other reproduction or redistribution is strictly prohibited. All rights reserved.

- Warranty of merchantability: An implied warranty stating that the product or item is fit for the purpose intended by the manufacturer.
- Implied warranty of fitness for a particular purpose: An implied warranty that a product or item is fit for a specific purpose about which the seller is informed or for which the seller recommends the product.
- Disclaimer: A manufacturer or individual's refusal to respect a warranty. The Uniform Commercial Code designates actions to be taken to disclaim a warranty. However, if a warranty and disclaimer are both contained in the same communication, the disclaimer is not enforceable.
- Statutes of repose: A statute of limitation based upon the date of sale as opposed to the date the injury occurred. This limitation protects manufacturers from frivolous claims about products (e.g., an injury occurring years after purchase and use of a product).
- Breach of warranty: A claim brought by a party stating that a product's warranty is false. This claim is much like a breach of contract claim. Normally, punitive damages are not applicable to this type of claim.

Parallels between product liability and toxic tort claims

Product liability laws and toxic tort laws can meet in that a claimant's toxic exposure may require remedy under strict liability in a tort action. Also, the claimant's exposure may appear similar to a product liability action if the party has worked with a toxic product or had been exposed to the product at his/her place of employment. Recently, manufacturer strict liability has been added to product liability theories. Under this liability, the plaintiff does not have to prove fault or intent, but he/she does have to prove the product was unduly dangerous because of a defect, the defect was present in the product at the time it left the manufacturer's control, and there is a causal relationship between the injury and the defect. Thus, a party's complaint may contain counts of negligence and strict liability.

Restatement (Second) of Torts, Sec. 402A (1965)

The section provides that, "One who sells any product in a defective condition, unreasonably dangerous to the user or consumer or to his property, is subject to liability for physical harm thereby caused to the ultimate user or consumer, or his property, if: (A)

Copyright © Mometrix Media. You have been licensed one copy of this document for personal use only. Any other reproduction or redistribution is strictly prohibited. All rights reserved.

the seller is engaged in the business of selling such a product, and (B) the product is expected to and does reach the user or consumer without substantial change in the condition in which it is sold." Thus, the manufacturer is responsible to the public for injuries that may be caused by a product manufactured for profit. In product liability law, there are three causes of action. These causes encompass strict liability, negligence, and breach of contract.

Copyright © Mometrix Media. You have been licensed one copy of this document for personal use only.
Any other reproduction or redistribution is strictly prohibited. All rights reserved.

Workers' Compensation

Role of the LNC as a Workers' Compensation Manager

There are two primary goals for the Workers' Compensation Manager. First is the coordination, implementation, and evaluation of a claimant's needs. This process includes the LNC exercising cost-effective measures. The second goal is the return to work of the injured claimant. In addition to the two primary goals, the LNC as Workers' Compensation Manager, may negotiate rates for services, perform on-site audits to determine that billed services actually occurred, survey medical records, prepare rate evaluations, and attend defense medical examinations. The LNC may also perform an on-site evaluation of the work setting, which can include the structural make-up of the site, the job functions expected, and the physical requirements that may be demanded of the claimant. This onsite evaluation aids in determination of a timetable for return of claimant to the work place. All information obtained will be reported to attending medical personnel to aid in claimant's return to work.

Medical examinations

The independent medical examination and defense medical examination refer to the medical examination of a claimant in a workers' compensation claim. The counsel for plaintiff and the defense may agree upon the examiner to perform the claimant's evaluation, although the defense counsel has the right to choose the evaluating examiner. The LNC may attend the examination as an attorney representative. The LNC should prepare for the examination by becoming familiar with the specific medical claims, clarifying his/her level of participation, and the type of examination. Roles may vary. The LNC as case manager may attend to ask questions of the examining physician. The LNC as workers' compensation manager may attend strictly to observe. In addition, the case manager reviews the examiner's report to determine that all relevant questions are answered (Iyer 519). The LNC also maintains a written log of the examination procedures from entry to exit, preparing a report after the examination from the notes taken.

Copyright © Mometrix Media. You have been licensed one copy of this document for personal use only. Any other reproduction or redistribution is strictly prohibited. All rights reserved.

Court testimony of the LNC

The LNC serves as a fact witness, rather than as an expert witness. The LNC's testimony will cover the observations made in the original report. The LNC may also testify regarding observations made at the actual examination, if the LNC was present and can accurately recall the events. The attorney questioning the LNC may request he/she read the report into the record. The LNC, at all times during testimony, shall recall the events of the examination, but not judge the examination. In the event of a conflict between the LNC's report and the examiner's report, the LNC will report only the events he/she saw and heard, not interpret the examination report or determine the cause of discrepancies/

Workers' compensation claim

Although the claimant in a workers' compensation action may resolve the claim for lost wages, the case may remain open due to continued medical expenses. If the injured worker is unable to return to work or will require continued medical care, the nurse case manager may have to oversee the treatment. When continued care is required, the worker likely suffered a permanent or catastrophic injury. In these instances, the nurse case manager will attempt to refer long-term care actions to vocational rehabilitation. When long-term care is required, the nurse case manager will have to monitor the workers' care relative to prevention of complications. When traumatic brain injury occurs, the nurse case manager may have to work with family members and attend team meetings to aid in care facility decisions.

Purpose of workers' compensation insurance

Workers' compensation insurance is designed to cover an employee during the course of, and in the scope of, employment. The coverage is required pursuant to state regulations. States outline covered services and payments that employers must maintain to provide care for injured workers, as well as benefits for dependents in the event of a work-related death. The coverage is designed to provide both medical and wage benefits. The insurance is maintained under a no-fault system, and the employer is responsible for occupational injuries and damages no matter which party is found at fault for untoward occurrences and resultant damages. The state where the injured worker resides retains jurisdiction of the workers' compensation claim.

Copyright © Mometrix Media. You have been licensed one copy of this document for personal use only. Any other reproduction or redistribution is strictly prohibited. All rights reserved.

LNC's role in workers' compensation claims

Because work-related injuries can be permanent and catastrophic, workers' compensation is an important area of knowledge for the LNC. Currently, this area of practice is one of the most common for LNCs. The LNC may have to work closely with financial or employment consultants in an effort to determine lost wages, future costs, and any lifetime reserves the worker may require. Because each state and/or federal government maintains its own laws regarding workers' compensation benefits, the LNC should be knowledgeable about the laws in the state in which he/she practices. Most work-related compensatory programs function in a specific order. First, the injury/illness as a result of the workplace or job will occur. Second, the employee will report the injury/illness to the appropriate employment representative. Third, the employer will notify the claim department or insurance representative of the report. Fourth, the claims department will review the incident to determine whether compensation is applicable, will advise pertinent parties of the determination, and will adjudicate the action. Last, the department will monitor the claim and pay expenses as required.

Disagreement regarding compensation

When the injured employee and the insurance company are unable to agree regarding compensation, a hearing is requested. The hearing is requested through a formal document filed with the industrial commission or board maintaining jurisdiction. The board's commissioner will be a state-appointed official. This official will review all workers' compensation claims. A hearing will be scheduled and heard before the commissioner. Both parties will submit evidence, and the commissioner will make a determination based upon the evidence. If the commissioner determines the claim is a work-related injury, all parties to the action must inform the board of progress through reports filed as required by the commission. The employee's return to work, conclusion of benefits, or settlement will result in the filing being closed.

Copyright © Mometrix Media. You have been licensed one copy of this document for personal use only.
Any other reproduction or redistribution is strictly prohibited. All rights reserved.

Medical Documentation

Definitions

- Documentation: This applies all relevant information regarding a patient's care placed in the medical record.
- Health information: This applies to the information a health care provider, health plan, employer, life insurer, school, public health authority, or health care clearinghouse creates or receives.
- Quality assurance: The procedure designed to evaluate patient care provided by a health care provider. The records are reviewed to make changes for better patient care.
- Continuous quality improvement: This procedure supplements quality assurance, granting that work groups are the experts and should utilized to determine quality, problems, and solutions. The input provided is then utilized to confirm and analyze problems, measure improvement, and compliance with appropriate standards of care.
- Risk management: This is a quality assurance procedure to aid in the prevention of financial loss through patient, staff, and visitor claims. This procedure involves identification and analysis of problems prior to occurrence.
- Narrative charting: This chart is a narrative paragraph describing a patient's status, treatment, medication, and relevant information.
- Problem-oriented charting: This allows all health care team members to chart information relative to the problems a patient experiences, as well as the plan of care. This method utilizes the SOAP and SOAPIE formats.
- PIE charting: This problem-oriented procedure comprises progress notes, assessment, and patient care flow sheets. PIE stands for Problems, Intervention, and Evaluation of Nursing Care.
- Focus charting: This procedure arranges narrative documents for each consideration by diagnosis, action, response, and teaching. Rather than use the term "problem" for patient concerns, this charting uses the term "focus."
- Charting by exception (CBE): This charting maintains only abnormal findings and documents pertaining to standards of practice.

Copyright © Mometrix Media. You have been licensed one copy of this document for personal use only. Any other reproduction or redistribution is strictly prohibited. All rights reserved.

- Clinical pathway: This charting is event oriented, providing a multidisciplinary device to foresee disease outcomes, problems, and interventions.
- Electronic charting: This form of charting is by use of computer.
- Electronic documentation: This system utilizes computer hardware and software designed for a specific purpose to collect, process, sort, store, print, and display data produced through health care delivery to patients.
- Computer hardware: This hardware provides the interface to let the health care provider enter and obtain information. This may involve a single personal computer designed for a single purpose, or it may involve several personal computers creating a network.
- Computer software: This software is designed to tell the computer hardware what, when, and how to accomplish a task. The instructions designed may be simple or more involved.
- Physical security: When utilizing electronic documentation, this security refers to protection of information by unauthorized individuals.
- Personnel security: This security pertains to prudent selection of individuals who will be able to access confidential information. Strict adherence to this security procedure can reduce the chance of breach of confidentiality.
- System security: This brings together both physical security and personnel security to insure information within the electronic system remains confidential and secure. The security generally involves institutional polices for protection.
- Encryption: To prevent any individual from obtaining and reading electronic information, the data is manipulated.
- Audit trail: This "trail" is designed as a record of all individuals who have accessed each record and when accessed.

Purposes

The main purpose in documenting medical information is to recognize patient status, the need for care, and the plan to deliver and evaluate the care. Some additional purposes include a record of personal health protection, cost-benefit reduction documentation, and risk management. Evidence of compliance with standards, rules, regulations, and laws for health care practices is also contained in the record. Student learning experience information can be gained from records. The patient's rights are documented in the records, as is professional and ethical conduct of each health care provider. Information

Copyright © Mometrix Media. You have been licensed one copy of this document for personal use only. Any other reproduction or redistribution is strictly prohibited. All rights reserved.

regarding care required on discharge and for future health care will be contained in the record. The record also provides appropriate information for billing and insurance reimbursement purposes. The Joint Commission on Accreditation for Healthcare Organizations, as well as federal and state agencies, can review records for evaluation.

Failure to maintain records and confidentiality of patient records

The nurse's best defense in any legal action is factual and thorough recording. Nurses who do not document patient care normally indicate a lack of time as the reason. Though this may be the case, it is not an exemption from legal and disciplinary action. Documentation that does not contact adequate information can also impact a nurse in a negative fashion, even if he/she provided excellent care. The institution for whom the information is recorded should assume responsibility to insure the patient records are complete. In addition, the nurse should be aware of the legal, ethical, employment and social implications of patient confidentiality. The Health Insurance Portability and Accountability Act (HIPAA) (1996) is designed to protect patient record privacy. The nurse should also be aware of an institution's policies regarding faxing medical records and patient information, since this information must remain confidential. The nurse should be aware of the type of information that can be faxed.

Narrative charting

Advantages: This is the most common form of documentation, so it is familiar and comfortable to health care providers. This method can be combined with other methods without problems. The chronological events can be recorded effortlessly, and the patient's status interventions, treatment, and responses to treatment are documented.

Disadvantages: Since handwritten, the writing may not be legible. Sometimes, too much information or not enough information is contained in the record. The information may be disorganized and recording can be time-consuming. The lack of information in the record may be related to the nursing process and demonstration of critical thinking, analysis, and decision making.

Copyright © Mometrix Media. You have been licensed one copy of this document for personal use only.
Any other reproduction or redistribution is strictly prohibited. All rights reserved.

SOAP and SOAPIE formats

SOAP format involves subjective data, objective data, assessment, and plan. SOAPIE format encompasses subjective data, objective data, assessment, plan, interventions, and evaluation.

Advantages: This chart is organized in a particular format, allowing for easier monitoring of issues that arise. The problems can be numbered for rapid reference for use with care plans. The nursing process is exhibited in this record, and communication between health care providers is improved. Discharge summaries and resolution (if applicable) are noted. If problems are not resolved, the record contains notes for treatment and the procedure to distribute this information among applicable health care providers.

Disadvantages: This format requires nurses to re-learn the procedure to apply information into the appropriate SOAP or SOAPIE plan, which can result in blanks when the nurse cannot determine proper categorization and time-consuming efforts. The plan may also cause repetitious information in the record. Health care providers may also resist implementation of this process.

PIE charting

Advantages: This format streamlines charting, decreases repetition, and deletes the separate care plan. Since the nurse records evaluation of problems he/she has identified during each shift, continuing care is guaranteed. The format also enhances the merit of progress notes and works effectively in both primary nursing and psychiatric settings.

Disadvantages: Since nurses record evaluations during each shift, the chart can become lengthy. Staffing mix may cause issues since the care planning is the RN's duty. The chart may not appropriate address patient outcomes, and it may not be appropriate for those patients who do not have changing problems. Also, since no practice guidelines, care plans, or clinical paths exist, discrepancies may arise.

Copyright © Mometrix Media. You have been licensed one copy of this document for personal use only.
Any other reproduction or redistribution is strictly prohibited. All rights reserved.

Focus charting

Advantages: The patient's response is included, identifying concerns and needs. The nursing process is encouraged, including judgment and analytical thinking to ascertain patient status from the information in the record. Structured progress notes are developed. The focus column utilized makes patient information comprehensible.

Disadvantages: Incorporating and documenting notes on the content and focus may prove burdensome. The information must be ordered into categories of data, action, and patient response. If patient responses are not noted, the format may prove to be no more than narrative charting.

Charting by exception

Advantages: The charts contain easily accessible, up-to-date patient information comprised of SOAP notes, flow sheets, incidental order, protocols, standards of practice, and nursing diagnosis care plans. These flow sheets negate scratch notes. The form guidelines on the reverse side of charting documents assist nurses. The charting is not normally repetitious. The format identifies normal patient findings, and is adaptable to clinical pathways charting.

Disadvantages: Some repetitious charting does occur. The format is geared toward an all-RN staff. Documentation tools must be revised, and staff that is used to more comprehensive documenting systems must be re-educated. Routine activities are not documented, so reimbursement may be a factor. This format can pose a problem when defending a claim, since the charting tends to be intermittent, causing questions about detection of conditions and symptoms.

Electronic charting

Advantages: Electronic charting can provide precise and timely documentation, with simple access to patient information. The format provides effective communication, with legible information contained in the chart. Also, this format can aid in patient confidentiality.

Copyright © Mometrix Media. You have been licensed one copy of this document for personal use only. Any other reproduction or redistribution is strictly prohibited. All rights reserved.

Disadvantages: Although this form may aid in patient confidentiality, it can also pose increased risk in the same area. The downtime is greater. Health care providers may experience problems when converting to a paperless chart, and training is required, adding to the cost of the equipment. If not enough terminals are available, information may not be added timely. The staff may experience a false sense of security, believing the data contained in the chart is flawless. Downtime is experienced while institutions compare and consider software.

Legal and ethical issues

- Confidentiality: Institutions must address time limits for information to remain on-screen to avoid unattended records exposure; placing screens in low-traffic, low-access areas; determination of information regarding a person requesting sensitive information; password use; and limiting access to those individuals who need to obtain information.
- Employee access: Institutions must develop criteria for employee accessibility to records, notably how accessed, what can be accessed, and limited access for certain information.
- Patient privacy: Institutions must take all measures to protect patient and family privacy, especially from those who may abuse this charting format.
- Accuracy of data input: To insure accuracy and timeliness of records input, institutions must develop procedures for those utilizing the system. Employees' computer skills should be checked and training programs organized.
- Patient's right to a copy of record: Institutions must develop policies regarding release of computerized patient records when requested by a patient or his/her attorney.

HIPAA Rules for Standards for Privacy of Individually Identifiable Health Information

The Rules were published on December 28, 2000, to be complied with by April 14, 2003, or April 14, 2004 if a small health plan. The Rules apply to all health plans, all health care providers submitting health information in electronic form relative to a standard transaction, and all health care clearinghouses. The Rule has four purposes: (1) improve

Copyright © Mometrix Media. You have been licensed one copy of this document for personal use only. Any other reproduction or redistribution is strictly prohibited. All rights reserved.

and protect consumer rights through control of improper use of medical information, (2) provide each patient access to his/her information, (3) increase the quality of health care and trust by consumers, and (4) provide a framework of health care privacy protection on a national level.

Effective medical documentation

The elements of effective medical documentation include factual, accurate, complete, and timely information. Effective documentation provides a written record containing important facts for a chain of events over a specific period of time. The charts, records, and documents also require preparation and maintenance of the history of events. The entries should demonstrate the patient's care needs, problems, and a plan of action to fulfill the required care. Documentation should reflect the professional monitoring of a patient, including the nurse's judgment and actions, the patient's progress, and the results of care. Effective notes include the nurse's entry of all activities on behalf of the patient, as well as notes related to evaluation of care and treatment.

Importance of factual, accurate, complete, and timely information when documenting patient's records
- First, keep all documentation factual. In doing so, use specific and factual language, avoiding relative or vague statements. The words used by a patient to explain his/her symptoms should be noted as well.
- Second, keep all documentation accurate. The patient's name should be on every sheet in the chart/record. To that end, the nurse should always check the patient's name on the chart prior to making notations. The nurse should limit notations to those issues he/she has actually observed and should be sure to understand a medical term prior to using it in the chart. Spelling is important to avoid a lack of credibility. The nurse's medical knowledge should be up-to-date (e.g., terminology, new diseases) to be certain to chart information about which he/she has an understanding.
- Third, the records should be complete, including information that has been communicated to another health care provider. Last, the nurse should include the date of time of each chart entry, entries should be in chronological order, the entry

Copyright © Mometrix Media. You have been licensed one copy of this document for personal use only. Any other reproduction or redistribution is strictly prohibited. All rights reserved.

should not be made prior to care or backdated, and entries should be charted as soon as possible to avoid delay between entries.

Effective institutional policies and procedures relative to effective documentation

Obviously, the nurse should record all entries in accordance with the institution's approved regulations. The nurse should record entries only on the forms approved by the facility. The institution should maintain a set of abbreviations, and the nurse should follow those strictly to avoid misunderstandings or abbreviations that can indicate two separate conditions. The nurse's name/initials and title should appear with each entry, leaving no space between the signature and the last entry made. No blank lines should be left on the chart; instead, use 'NA' to indicate it is not applicable. The chart should not contain language considered slang, no chart entry should be erased, eliminated with correction fluid, or rewritten. Normally, institutions require black or blue ink for entries, which allows for better copies if needed. The charting should be limited to the facility's documents, avoiding post-in notes or other scraps stapled or clipped to the chart. The specific times of each treatment should be noted, as well as details regarding vital signs.

Effective documentation in special situations

- With telephone and verbal orders, the nurse should write the order and have it co-signed pursuant to institution policy and procedure. A do not resuscitate order via telephone is not recommended, but if done, the nurse and another witness must receive the order. The nurse must chart that both he/she and the witness heard the order.
- The medication, route, site, time, reason, nurse's name/initials, and patient response should be noted when giving medications. Controlled substance removal or discard requires following specific policies and procedures of the institution. This must be done to avoid redirection of drugs.
- Charting the reason for administration, site, time, and patient's response are necessary when documenting a controlled substance. Medication error reporting forms should note the type of event, facts, witnesses, date, time, location, person who discovered the issue, patient's status, the name and time of each person notified, the name and title of the individual completing the form, the date of the report, and the name of each person who receives a copy of the form.

Copyright © Mometrix Media. You have been licensed one copy of this document for personal use only. Any other reproduction or redistribution is strictly prohibited. All rights reserved.

<u>Effective charting when a patient leaves against medical advice</u>
The patient should be informed of all potential risks involved when leaving against medical advice. This information should be provided by an appropriate health care provider. The institution's attorney should prepare a form the patient should sign prior to leaving the facility. This form should indicate the patient has been informed of risks and dangers associated with leaving against medical advice. If the patient will not sign the form, the attending health care provider should document precisely what the patient was told and that he/she refused to sign. The patient's mental status should be charted as well, including his/her reason for leaving, as indicated by the patient. If family members or friends are present, this should be noted, including the fact that they have been notified of the risks of leaving and given care instructions. If the family members or friends are not present, but have been notified, this should be noted with details of discussion. Any follow-up or care instructions given to the patient should be charted. The patient's destination, method of transport, time of leave, mental and physical condition, and names of each person accompanying him/her should be documented.

DNR orders and discharge planning

- Each institution should maintain policies regarding do not resuscitate orders (DNR). The facility should review these policies periodically. It is advisable to place a time limit on this type of policy to insure periodic review. The do not resuscitate order must be charted to protect a health care provider from a potential medical malpractice lawsuit. The order should be noted, as well as details of discussions with the patient or family members. The facility should have a form stating what may happen when a patient is not resuscitated. The patient and/or family member consenting to the order should sign and date this form.
- When discharging a patient, it is essential the patient be aware that treatment and care will be discontinued, the date of discontinuance, the consequences, alternative resource, and a plan of action after the effective date. This information should be documented in detail, and a form should be signed and dated by the patient and/or family member with whom the health care provider discusses the discharge information.

Copyright © Mometrix Media. You have been licensed one copy of this document for personal use only. Any other reproduction or redistribution is strictly prohibited. All rights reserved.

Owner of patient's medical records

The medical facility is the owner of a patient's medical records. However, the patient may request copies of the records, at which point the facility must produce the records. Some states have laws regarding release of records, including time limits and reproduction costs. The medical records may be utilized in legal matters. In this case, the records may be requested by a plaintiff's attorney. The attorney may request records on behalf of a client prior to litigation, or the records may be requested through a subpoena duces tecum or request for production of documents after a lawsuit has been filed. The health records of an employee may be reviewed by outside agencies. These records should provide sufficient documentation without releasing privileged or confidential information. The OSHA Standard for Prevention of Transmission of Bloodborne Pathogens in the Workplace provides that test results relative to occupational exposure to HIB or HBV should be separate from the employee's personnel record. These results should not be released to attorneys pursuant to subpoenas directed to a health care provider's personnel or health file.

Reportable incidents and forms

An incident is defined as an occurrence, accident, or event inconsistent with an institution's normal care of a patient. Generally, these incidents include falls, medical errors or unexpected reactions, treatment errors, patient injuries caused by the patient (e.g., self-mutilation), patient wandering, eating or drinking substances outside the scope of medical care, abusive behavior toward staff or family or abusive behavior of family or other toward patient, complaints about treatment, personal property reported as stolen or missing, injuries sustained by visitors. When an incident occurs, an incident, variance, or occurrence report must be completed. The form should be completed by the health care provider with first-hand knowledge of the incident or an individual with second-hand knowledge of the occurrence (e.g., supervisor or nurse manager). Each state maintains laws regarding whether this form is discoverable during litigation.

Purpose of incident reports
An incident reporting system has been established by the Joint Commission. These forms provide necessary information to provide the best possible care to patients. The forms provide a means to determine problem areas, make assessment for in-service teaching, and

- 79 -

Copyright © Mometrix Media. You have been licensed one copy of this document for personal use only. Any other reproduction or redistribution is strictly prohibited. All rights reserved.

to reduce patient and family hazards. The form also assists in evaluation of health care providers and required changes in policies and procedures, if applicable. The risk management department of a facility will also utilize this form to determine whether changes are required in policies and procedures or potential exists for a lawsuit. The form may also help determine whether supplemental training or counseling may be needed for the nurse or other health care provider involved in the incident.

Legal and ethical issues of completing an incident report

A nurse should prepare an incident report only if he/she has first-hand knowledge of the events. Each occurrence must be reported, and a nurse who fails to do so could face termination of employment. In addition, a nurse may subject himself/herself to personal liability if the report is not filed and the incident results in harm or injury to a patient or another individual. A nurse has a professional and ethical responsibility to record the incident pursuant to institution policies. The report itself is considered an administrative record, rather than a portion of the medical record.

Documenting information when preparing an incident report

When reporting an incident defined as "reportable," the form should contain an area to write a brief factual description. The names, addresses, and telephone numbers of all witnesses should be included. The condition of the patient prior to the incident should be noted, as well as the condition (e.g., death) and attitude (e.g., angry) afterward. The report should note the last time the patient was seen and who saw him/her. The name, title, and department of the individual with first-hand knowledge of the incident must be noted, as well as any review by the department head or head nurse. The report should be signed and dated by the person preparing it, as well as by individual reviewing it. A comments section should be available, as well as specific questions to be answered (e.g., injury, treatment offered/refused/accepted, notification of physician, x-ray ordered). The report should also provide information regarding results of any tests as a result of the incident and intended follow-up.

Information that should be excluded from an incident report

The incident report should not contain information that could damage the institution. This information may include physician comments or orders. Also, a personal opinion or

- 80 -

Copyright © Mometrix Media. You have been licensed one copy of this document for personal use only. Any other reproduction or redistribution is strictly prohibited. All rights reserved.

judgmental conclusion regarding the incident need not be included. No indication regarding an assumption of the responsible party should be made. The form should not include recommended improvements, different procedures that could be followed, or thoughts regarding prevention of a repeat occurrence. Witness statements are not included in the report, nor are the facility's actions to correct the issue. Indication of copies distributed to other parties, any evaluations done as a result of the incident, or accusations are not necessary. No admissions should be included in the report. One report should be prepared, combining witness reports.

Individuals or committees who may review the incident report

The report may be read by several individuals or committees to grant evaluation and investigation of the incident. The nurse who witnessed the incident and the nursing head or supervisor will read the report. The attending physician may read the report. Administrative officials, quality assurance department members, and risk management department members may review and evaluate the report. The facility's attorney, plaintiff's attorney (if allowable), and the facility's insurance company representative may review the information. As a result of the incident, several actions will take place. The witnessing nurse must document the incident in an incident report, as well as provide factual information in the medical record. The nurse supervisor or department head will receive a copy of the report, as well as appropriate administrative staff. The report will be forwarded to specific departments or individuals for review and possible follow-up. After review by appropriate departments or individuals, modifications may be recommended that might include policy changes, personnel changes, additional education or training, or reprimands or employment termination.

Electronic documentation

Confidentiality

The Health Insurance Portability and Accountability Act, the American Medical Association, the American Nurses Association, and the Joint Commission on Accreditation of Healthcare Organizations require and/or emphasize that maintenance of patient confidentiality is essential. However, some information can be shared under certain circumstances. Some of these instances may include providing information to another health care provider to supplement a patient's diagnosis and treatment; use of information for educational

Copyright © Mometrix Media. You have been licensed one copy of this document for personal use only.
Any other reproduction or redistribution is strictly prohibited. All rights reserved.

purposes; use of information for health care audits, evaluations, and peer review (without disclosing a patient's identity). Electronic documentation increases the possibility of breach of confidentiality because of user ability to access, transmit, and copy information. Increasing the security of records while maintaining the health care provider's need for information to provide care can be addressed through physical security, personnel security, and system security approaches.

Threats to physical security

Three possible threats exist in relation to the physical security of electronic documentation. The physical security of the system involves protection from access by unauthorized persons. First, the video displays and personal computers may be placed in an area that allows unauthorized individuals to view information. The placement of the system must be such that authorized personnel can view and enter information, but that prevents unauthorized individuals from doing so. Second, the stored information must be placed to avoid theft of data storage devices. Information on the hard drive can be transferred to a diskette or CD-ROM or the computer can be picked up by an unauthorized individual. These incidents will cause a breach of confidentiality and should be avoided by transferring and storing information in a secure, remote location; modifying hard disk drives so information cannot be copied; and properly securing hardware and computers to avoid theft. Third, information cannot be damage or lost due to power surges, fire, floods, or other like occurrences.

Personnel security

First, employees entitled to access information should be carefully selected. After employees are selected, each must be properly trained to use the equipment, which should include procedures to conserve confidentiality, appropriate use of the system and hardware, and knowledge of disciplinary actions to which he/she will be subject in the event of a breach. Once training is completed, it should be documented and the employee should sign a statement of agreement regarding confidentiality practices. Passwords or sign-on codes will also aid in personnel security. If an individual without a valid password attempts entry, the system will not allow entry into records. Passwords also identify each user and can limit each user to certain sections of the system. The system can also be equipped with software designed to delete a user's password after a specified period of inactivity.

Copyright © Mometrix Media. You have been licensed one copy of this document for personal use only. Any other reproduction or redistribution is strictly prohibited. All rights reserved.

System security

To ensure system security, the personnel security and physical security are combined to maintain a multilevel system maintaining confidentiality. Normally, the facility institutes policies to protect the documentation system. The policies may encompass the type and amount of data that can be collected, classification of employees that may be given passwords or sign-on codes, or a system that includes the issue, tracking, and deletion of authorized passwords or sign-on codes. The computer system should also be protected from viruses and should include careful monitoring of any occurrence that may risk a security breach. The institution should also maintain a policy for backing up data. The system may also contain an encryption code or an audit trail.

Considerations of electronic documentation integrity

The authenticity of the data is an important element when maintaining the integrity of a system. The information should be identical to that originally entered by an individual. Ordinarily, the system will allow a user to review material before it is added to a patient's electronic chart. If the user wishes to revise the information, modification can be achieves prior to adding the data to the patient's record. The system may also compare the information to be input with a set of input requirements. The system may require that the information comply wit the input requirements before accepting it. Errors can usually be corrected after the information has been added if the user utilizes an error removal mechanism combined with the audit trail. Integrity is also maintained by use of individual identification, normally through passwords.

Advantages

If a system is well-designed, it can improve the care given to patients, save an institution time and money, and advance interdisciplinary care. Nurse overtime can be reduced through preformatted or standardized electronic documentation. Also, through proper coding, one piece of information can prompt several activities. Medical information can be obtained quickly, allowing efficient notice of abnormal tests or rapid retrieval of diagnostic information. Trends in a patient's reaction or behavior can be detected and programs may be designed to remind health care providers of possible patient problems. These can all result in improved patient care and treatment. Documentation is also legible and maintained in an orderly manner. The system can also group information together, allowing all caregivers easy access to necessary information.

Copyright © Mometrix Media. You have been licensed one copy of this document for personal use only. Any other reproduction or redistribution is strictly prohibited. All rights reserved.

Common problems

The institution must be committed to the electronic system; otherwise, the documentation and information in the system may be fragmented. This fragmentation will result in the inability of health care providers to determine patient care received and patient response to the care. The institution must also be aware of the number of terminals needed to allow effective electronic charting, as well as placement in a location that allows users to readily input data. Those individuals who need to review data must also be able to access the information easily, rather than having to wait for print-outs or terminals. Computer downtime is a drawback that interferes with documentation input or access. The system must be designed to consider the needs and uses of several types of health care providers. The time needed to acquaint users with the system and the type of data it will provide can also result in an initial time increase to become familiar with the system. Obviously, errors can occur, despite all precautions. Also, duplication in charting can occur if a health care provider does not have faith in the system and, therefore, charts electronically and on paper.

Copyright © Mometrix Media. You have been licensed one copy of this document for personal use only. Any other reproduction or redistribution is strictly prohibited. All rights reserved.

Informed Consent

When an informed consent is required

Generally, the informed consent is needed whenever a health care provider intends to touch a patient. A consent to treatment form is normally signed by the patient when he/she is admitted to an institution. This form is designed to allow the facility to perform routine procedures or treatment. "Routine" generally implies those procedures that are basically noninvasive and for which there is low risk of injury. On the other hand, a surgical procedure normally requires a specific informed consent and confirming documentation showing the consent was properly obtained. If the patient will be subject to procedures that have material risks, complications, or consequences that may impact a patient, an informed consent is needed. Generally, a patient must be properly informed to make decisions when he/she may be subject to a health risk during treatment.

General criteria of capacity to consent

A person who consents to or refuses treatment must be legally capable of doing so; he/she must have the legal capacity to make the decision. In other words, he/she must be able to understand the nature and effects of his/her acts. Courts normally interpret a person's capacity when in question. Normally, the courts will presume a person is competent, unless he/she has been proven incompetent. In the case of decision-making capacity, a person have the ability to participate in his/her care and treatment decisions if he/she understands the medical condition, pertinent information is presented to the patient, and the patient is able to communicate preferred treatment and the reason for same. If a person is incapable of making health care decisions, a legal representative may do so. In most states, the durable power of attorney statutes grant individuals the power to appoint a representative while still able to do so. This representative is granted the authority to make decisions when the patient cannot. The probate court may appoint a guardian or advocate to make decisions if a representative has not been appointed by the patient prior to incompetence.

Copyright © Mometrix Media. You have been licensed one copy of this document for personal use only. Any other reproduction or redistribution is strictly prohibited. All rights reserved.

Express consent and implied consent

Expressed consent is consent actually given by a patient either verbally or in writing. Implied consent involves care in emergency situations or when a patient's actions may indicate a presumption that treatment should proceed. If the patient does not waive consent or implied consent is not present, the health care provider must obtain the patient's informed consent. The best procedure is to have a patient sign a consent-to-treatment form when proposed treatment is discussed. The nurse should be certain that the patient has been informed of treatment and that all questions are answered. If the nurse finds that a patient's has not been properly informed or questions answered, the nurse should take measures to ensure the health care provider performs this duty. In medical emergencies, the law does not necessarily require informed consent. When it is not possible to obtain informed consent, the law assumes the patient would consent under the doctrine of implied consent. Implied consent may also apply when a patient voluntarily visits a clinic or physician's office.

Nurse's role

Nurses may sign as witnesses to an informed consent. The nurse is not obtaining the consent, but is simply acting as a witness to the signature of the form. The nurse is not responsible for verification of information and should not indicate responsibility on the form, unless he/she has been present when it was given. The health care provider is responsible for informed consent, unless the nurse provides answers to questions that would otherwise be answered by a health care provider. The nurse should refer these questions to the treating physician. The nurse does not assume the provider's duty regarding information presented to the patient, but may support same. Informed consent is considered proper when a written and signed and the health care provider has noted the discussion and consent in the chart. The patient must prove the consent was obtained through fraud or bad faith to invalidate it. If a patient cannot understand English, the health care provider should provide a translator.

Health care provider's duty to disclose when obtaining

The health care provider must disclose to the patient certain information when obtaining an informed consent for a treatment or procedure. The duty to disclose includes the name

Copyright © Mometrix Media. You have been licensed one copy of this document for personal use only. Any other reproduction or redistribution is strictly prohibited. All rights reserved.

of the person(s) providing the treatment. The patient must be informed of the health care provider's diagnosis. The health care provider must notify the patient of all conflicts of interest that may exist. The nature and purpose of the treatment, possible consequences and risks associated with the treatment, and anticipated benefits of treatment must be discussed. Also, the patient must be informed of any other options that may exist, as well as any anticipated consequences if he/she does not receive the treatment.

Exceptions to the duty to disclose

Although exceptions to the duty to disclose do exist, they vary from state to state. To prevent medical malpractice liability, the reasons for not informing a patient should be carefully documented. Two basic rules apply relative to the physician's duty to disclose. First, the physician should disclose information similar to that which would be disclosed by others in the medical community under similar circumstances. Second, and less accepted, is patient-oriented and deals with the actual information a reasonable patient would require in order to make an informed decision. Normally, the exceptions to the duty to disclose include emergencies, a patient's waiver of right to receive the information, the therapeutic privilege when a physician believes the information may be harmful to the patient, obvious risk, and a public health requirement.

Minors

Each state maintains an age of majority. Any person younger than the age of majority is considered a minor. An emancipated minor must be financially independent, reside apart from his/her parents, be married, be in the military service of the United States, or be considered to have the legal capacity of an adult. If the court determines a minor thoroughly understands the character and effect of a proposed treatment, even if that minor is of a young age, he/she may be declared a mature minor able to make a medical decision. There are exceptions to parent consent when a minor is involved in medical treatment decisions; these exceptions vary by state. In some instances, a minor is able to make medical decisions involving sexually transmitted diseases, pregnancy-related issues, and physical or substance abuse. The minor may also be entitled to make a decision in an emergency situation, or if he/she is declared emancipated or mature.

Copyright © Mometrix Media. You have been licensed one copy of this document for personal use only.
Any other reproduction or redistribution is strictly prohibited. All rights reserved.

Medical community and prudent patient standards

Courts utilize two standards when deciding informed consent actions, the medical community standard and the prudent patient standard. The medical community standard provides that the circumstances and general practices of the profession in similar matters dictates the physician's responsibility to inform a patient. In this case, the standard rests with the medical community. That plaintiff must prove the physician failed to provide information that a reasonable physician would have provided in a similar situation, resulting in injury to the patient. The prudent patient standard, also known as the material risk standard, provides that a reasonable individual is able to consider the risks involved in treatment. In this instance, the standard rests with the patient. The jury will determine whether the risk and possible harm would be considered by a reasonable person. The general idea of the prudent patient standard is that each patient has the right to make his/her decisions.

Considerations for nurses, physicians, and physician's assistants

The health care provider obtaining informed consent should consider several tips. The health care provider and the institution where employed should have a specific policy for informed consent. The health care provider should always be truthful about his/her qualifications. Health care providers obtaining consent should be aware of the requirements of the Board of Licensure and other professional agencies, as well as the requirements that may vary relative to office and surgery practices. Patients should be thoroughly informed; the health care provider can utilize literature, videotapes, and conferences to insure information reaches a patient. The treatment and options should be explained in layperson's language to insure understanding. The patient should be thoroughly informed of prescription drug dangers, including side effects, reactions, combination effects, and contraindications.

Liability without patient consent

A patient may claim that a health care provider is liable for damages as a result of assault and/or battery when informed consent has not been obtained. Assault is claimed when one person intentionally acts in a manner that another fears will result in being touched offensively or injuriously. In this instance, the first person does not actually have to touch

Copyright © Mometrix Media. You have been licensed one copy of this document for personal use only.
Any other reproduction or redistribution is strictly prohibited. All rights reserved.

the other. On the other hand, battery results when physical contact or touching actually occurs. Health care providers must obtain information consent prior to performing tests or providing treatment. Otherwise, the patient may claim the health care provider is guilty of assault or battery. The patient does not have to incur harm or injury to make this claim. The claimant must prove that informed consent was not given or that the health care provider performed beyond the range of the consent of the patient.

Negligently obtained informed consent

Professional negligence is likely to be the basis for a claim of treatment without informed consent. In this instance, the plaintiff must prove the claim through testimony of an expert witness. The claimant will be required to prove the health care provider failed to provide sufficient or appropriate information and breached his/her duty to the patient. Also, the claimant must prove that he/she would have made a different decision if more or appropriate information had been provided. Thus, the plaintiff's claim is that the injury was the result of the breach of duty.

Lack of consent action

The laws applied to lack of consent claims differ in each state. The courts may subject the action to a subjective standard or an objective standard. If utilizing the subject standard, the court will examine the circumstances and the actions of the plaintiff in the situation. Most courts do not review the decisions of the specific plaintiff in the action. Most courts review the claim under the objective standard. In this case, the courts will determine the actions of a "reasonable" individual when making medical decisions in a particular situation. Pursuant to the objective standard, a claimant may be required to prove that he/she was subjected to a risk not known to him/her, that the physician failed to disclose this risk, that a reasonable individual would have made a different decision if the risk had been known, and that injury resulted.

<u>Similarities and differences between subjective and objective standards</u>
Both standards require that a health care provider has a responsibility (duty) to provide certain information to a patient. If the health care provider fails to disclose information to a patient, the claimant may allege a breach of duty. The standards differ in the manner in which the courts view plaintiff's required proofs. The subjective standard requires plaintiff

Copyright © Mometrix Media. You have been licensed one copy of this document for personal use only. Any other reproduction or redistribution is strictly prohibited. All rights reserved.

to show only that treatment would have been refused if proper information ad been provided by the health care provider. The objective standard requires plaintiff to show that any reasonable person in the situation at issue would have refused treatment if all risks, benefits, and options had been explained.

Advance directives

Advance directives are designed to allow a competent individual to execute a document that provides control over his/her future care. These documents are known as living wills or durable powers of attorney for health care. The living will allows the individual to provide direction relative to his/her future health care and the care that can be accepted or refused. The living will is normally executed in the same manner as a last will and testament. The durable power of attorney for health care appoints an individual (the attorney-in-fact) who can make decisions on behalf of the principal (a competent adult) if he/she is declared incompetent in the future. The attorney-in-fact must receive the same information the principal would receive when making a medical decision on his/her behalf. Each state has laws allowing living wills or durable powers of attorney for health care to be executed, and health care providers are bound by the documents. The Patient Self-Determination Act of 1990 grants that all institutions receiving Medicare or Medicaid funds must advice patients of the right to refuse treatment and of all pertinent laws relative to advance directives.

Health care agents

Although called by different names, the legal documents that designate health care agents provide the same assurance of care in the event an individual is declared incompetent. State laws normally dictate the name and type of form. The forms can be known as "durable power of attorney for health care" or "health care representative form." The names also include "medical durable power of attorney," medical power of attorney," or "proxy appointment." Obviously, all health care providers should be aware of the different names for each form and the specific purpose of each form.

Copyright © Mometrix Media. You have been licensed one copy of this document for personal use only. Any other reproduction or redistribution is strictly prohibited. All rights reserved.

Euthanasia

The term euthanasia is meant to imply "good death." A patient should be granted a basically pain-free death when euthanasia applies. There are four types of euthanasia. First, a patient's consent is termed "voluntary." Second, if a patient is unable to consent or has not consented, but it is presumed he/she wishes to die, the euthanasia may be "involuntary." Third, when steps or actions are initiated that will result in the patient's death, an "active" euthanasia occurs. Fourth, "passive" euthanasia results when no action is taken to advance the patient's death.

Artificial nutrition and hydration

Both artificial nutrition and hydration provide life-sustaining treatments. These procedures provide a chemically balanced mix of nutrients and fluids which are given to the patient. The 'feeding' procedure utilized is through a tube placed into the patient's stomach, intestines, or veins. When making a decision regarding artificial nutrition and hydration, the health care provider must be knowledgeable about the policies and procedures required by the institution. The treatment may be ethically and legally discontinued under two circumstances. First, the patient may refuse treatment, but must be competent when doing so. Second, no benefit must exist to continue treatment.

Copyright © Mometrix Media. You have been licensed one copy of this document for personal use only. Any other reproduction or redistribution is strictly prohibited. All rights reserved.

Legal Terminology

- Actions at law: This type of civil lawsuit that granted a money award as part of the relief requested.

- Actions in equity: This type of civil lawsuit involves arguments where a money award will not preserve the damaged/injured party.

- Adjudication: This is the procedure to reach a judicial decision.

- Administrative law: This type of law surrounds those regulations made by and ruling state and federal administrative agencies.

- Adverse event (AE): Any unexpected modification of a patient's medical condition, including changes in a pre-existing condition. This event relates to changes during a study from the date of informed consent to study completion. The event does not have to be related to the drug or device that was part of the study.

- Affidavit: This document encompasses statements of fact by a party. The affidavit is signed voluntarily, under oath.

- Affirmative defense: Affirmative defenses are specific defenses to a plaintiff's claim.

- AHCPR: This is the Agency for Health Care Policy and Research. The agency sets practice standards relative to various patient care matters.

- AHRQ: This is the Agency for Healthcare Research and Quality. This agency was formerly the Agency for Health Care Policy and Research.

- Alternative dispute resolution: This allows for resolution of claims/disputes without the necessity of trial.

- Ambulance chasing: A term used to identify an action that takes advantage of individuals involved in a crisis. This form of action is unethical and negative.

- ANA: This is the American Nurses Association. The organization is the nurses association at the national level.

- Annotation: This type of writing is an essay that completely analyzes a certain legal rule.

- Appellant: An appellant files the appeal of another court verdict.

- Appellate jurisdiction: This jurisdiction grants a court the authority to review the rulings of other courts.

- Appellee: An appellee responds to the appeal filed by the appellant.

Copyright © Mometrix Media. You have been licensed one copy of this document for personal use only. Any other reproduction or redistribution is strictly prohibited. All rights reserved.

- Arraignment: The arraignment is the formal hearing that occurs to read charges to an accused party, and the party then enters his/her plea to the charges.
- ASCII: The acronym is the American Standard Code for Information Interchange. The code represents English characters as numbers and is utilized by many computer programs for transfer of text between computers.
- Assessment: In the nursing process, the first step wherein data is assembled and reviewed to prepare for diagnosis. In the LNC process, the information gathered for review relative to claims.
- Assigned risk: This type of risk is one that insurance underwriters balk at insuring. However, state law or other regulations may require the risk be insured. In that case, a pool of handlers each takes turns covering the risk.
- Attorney work product: These encompass the theories, conclusions, and working documents that an attorney prepares for the benefit of his/her client.
- Attorney-client privilege: This privilege involves confidentiality of communication between an attorney and client relative to legal advice and representation. Pursuant to this protection, the client may refuse to disclose confidential communications, as well as present anyone else from doing so.
- Autonomy: This refers to personal freedom and the right for each individual to make his/her own decisions to serve his/her best interest.
- Bail: To ensure that an accused party appears for trial, he/she is required to post this amount of money.
- Bench trial: This type of trial occurs without a jury.
- Beneficence: Beneficence relates to an ethical viewpoint. This view is that actions taken should be for the protection of the patient, including treatment that furthers health.
- Bill of particulars: The bill of particulars is a written, legal document that specifies the defendant's negligence and the damages claimed by plaintiff.
- Biomechanics: This science relates to the body's mechanics and its responses to different forces.
- Bond: A bond is required by a court when a conservator is appointed. The bond is designed to guarantee no losses to the estate if the conservator fails to properly manage, or unlawfully takes, the assets. If losses occur, the bonding agency provides reimbursement to the estate, and the bonding company may file suit to collect against the conservator.

Copyright © Mometrix Media. You have been licensed one copy of this document for personal use only. Any other reproduction or redistribution is strictly prohibited. All rights reserved.

- Book of business: This designates the particular forms of insurance products an insurance company might offer (e.g., automobile, health, and homeowners).
- Brief: This document is presented to the court to outline a party's alleged facts and law.
- Capitation: This type of health care coverage provides a specified amount per individual member for health care to be provided by a primary health care provider. The provider is then paid the specified amount on a periodic basis (e.g., monthly). The health care provider is paid even if no services are provided during the specified period.
- Carrier: This is the insurance company that provides an insurance policy or coverage.
- Case brief: This document is a report outlining a court's opinion.
- Case law: This document is prepared by the court and is an opinion that creates or interprets law.
- Case reporters: These books encompass the decisions of the courts.
- Cause of action: The cause of action encompasses those proofs designed to support the components of a claim (e.g., malpractice) and then form the foundation for litigation.
- Certiorari: The procedure that asks for review of a action or decision by a discretionary appeals court.
- CFR: This is the Code of Federal Regulations. The Code contains all nursing home regulations.
- Circumstantial evidence: This involves evidence that leans toward a fact or incident.
- Claims consultant: This individual is the insurance company representative who investigates a claim and participates in negotiations in an effort to reach agreement relative to the amount of a claimant's loss or the liability of the insurer.
- Claims management: By utilizing claims management, the overall expense incurred as a result of claims can be significantly lowered.
- Claims processor: This individual is the insurance carrier's employee assigned the task of handling claims that are received from patients or providers.
- Claims specialist/adjuster: This individual is an independent agent or an insurance carrier employee assigned the task of investigating claims, allocating insurance reserves, and settling claims filed against the company's insured party.

Copyright © Mometrix Media. You have been licensed one copy of this document for personal use only. Any other reproduction or redistribution is strictly prohibited. All rights reserved.

- Closing arguments: Each attorney presents closing arguments summarizing the evidence presented in favor of his/her client during the course of trial.
- CMS 1500: This form was previously the HCFA 1500. The form is utilized as the claim form to submit charges for Medicare and Medicaid services.
- CMS: This organization is the Center for Medicare and Medicaid Services. The organization was previously the HCFA.
- CNA: This refers to a Certified Nursing Assistant. The CNA must have concluded standardized training for nursing home employment.
- Collaboration: Relative to a LNC, this term refers to his/her partnership with legal and health care professionals when requested.
- Collegiality: Relative to a LNC, this terms refers to his/her intellectual sharing and its contribution to peers and colleagues.
- Conciliation: This refers to resolution of a dispute between parties in an amicable manner.
- Concurrent jurisdiction: This type of jurisdiction allows that two or more courts possess the authority to grant a ruling or determination in one matter.
- Concurring opinion: This document is presented as an opinion by a judge concurring with the majority rule, but the agreement is based upon different reasoning.
- Conservatee: This individual has been adjudged by the court to be incapable of managing his/her financial affairs or unable to provide for his/her own care. A conservator is then appointed for this individual.
- Conservator of the Estate: This conservator is the individual or entity appointed by the court to manage financial affairs for another individual adjudged unable to manage his/her own affairs.
- Conservator of the Person: This conservator is the individual or entity appointed by the court to manage the care and protection of another individual adjudged unable to care for him/herself.
- Conservator: The conservator is the individual or entity appointed by the court to manage either personal care and/or financial affairs of another individual who has been adjudged incompetent.
- Contingency fee: This is an attorney fee that is based strictly on the positive outcome of a case and represents a percentage of the award recovered.

Copyright © Mometrix Media. You have been licensed one copy of this document for personal use only. Any other reproduction or redistribution is strictly prohibited. All rights reserved.

- Contract: A written document between two or more parties entered into voluntarily by each. This agreement is a legally binding document setting forth responsibilities for services or work to be performed over a specified period or reason.
- Co-payment: Under an insurance policy, this is the insured's shared expense for specific covered costs, usually determined on a percentage basis.
- Coverage: This refers to the assurance against losses designated pursuant to the terms and conditions of an insurance policy. This term is interchangeable with "insurance" or "protection."
- CPT: This is the Current Procedural Terminology. Health care providers utilize this system for descriptions and their 5-digit codes to report services and procedures.
- Cross-examination: This entails an adverse attorney's questioning of a witness (e.g., at deposition or trial).
- Cross-jurisdictional advocacy: This refers to the linking of law and health care models to reduce dispute and encourage change. The LNC is the individual who manages the intervention, which involves clients in different jurisdictions.
- Culture brokering: A process designed to bridge gaps and decrease dispute or effect change between people of different cultural backgrounds.
- Damage mitigation: This is a procedures or processes employed to decrease or restrict damages as a result of an incident.
- Declarant: An individual who makes a sworn statement or affirmation.
- Deductible: Under an insurance policy, this amount is pre-determined and must be paid by the insured toward medical expenses prior to the benefits under the policy becoming effective.
- Demonstrative evidence: Physical evidence (e.g., models) that offers to specific proof other than to broadly explain or simplify a factual matter.
- Derivative claim: A type of claim brought by the injured person's spouse, child, or parent claiming damages as a result of loss of companionship, loss of services, or expenses incurred.
- Descriptive word index: This index appears at the end of a series of legal books designed to assist in access of information relative to a law or statute.
- Descriptor: This refers to a word or phrase that illustrates an idea, concept, or subject.
- Designated nonparty: A party not named in a lawsuit, but found liable for all or part of the damages.

Copyright © Mometrix Media. You have been licensed one copy of this document for personal use only. Any other reproduction or redistribution is strictly prohibited. All rights reserved.

- Digests: Digests collect headnotes, then organize the same alphabetically by topic. The system assists in location of additional sources by a researcher.
- Direct evidence: This type of evidence is presented by a witness who has first-hand or personal knowledge of an incident or who actually observed an incident.
- Direct examination: This type of witness questioning is done by the attorney who called the witness.
- Directed verdict: When a party to an action does not demonstrate a cause of action based upon the evidence, the judge may grant this verdict in favor of the other party, upon motion filed by that party.
- Dispositive motions: This type of motion is brought by an attorney in a lawsuit to get rid of either part of or all of an action prior to trial.
- Dissenting opinion: This document is presented as an opinion by a judge disagreeing with the majority rule.
- Docket control order: A judge's order setting forth deadlines for discovery, pre-trial hearing, etc., in a cause of action.
- Docket number: This number is given to a lawsuit when initially filed with the court and is utilized throughout the course of litigation for identification.
- Docket: A court record containing the brief record of court proceedings from the filing of the action through conclusion.
- DRG: This is the Diagnosis Related Group. The system classifies patients by diagnosis and procedure, or, at times, by age and discharge status.
- DRI: This refers to the Defense Research Institute. This professional organization is comprised of attorneys who are employed primarily to defend claims.
- Drug formulary: There are two types of drug formularies, which constitute a list of a health plan's preferred medications. Open (voluntary) formularies encompass both formulary and non-formulary drugs, while the closed formulary related to drugs contained only in the formulary.
- EPO: This is an Exclusive Provider Organization, which is a Managed Care Organization with health care providers whose plan and membership is exclusive.
- Equitable remedies: In the case of an action that does not allow for money damages to protect the claimant from harm or injury, this type of relief is granted.
- Errata sheet: If corrections are made to the deposition transcript, this document sets forth each correction.

Copyright © Mometrix Media. You have been licensed one copy of this document for personal use only. Any other reproduction or redistribution is strictly prohibited. All rights reserved.

- Ethics: This issue explores right and wrong, including the values of each viewpoint and the effect of each pertaining to actual circumstances. The LNC should utilize the ANA Code for Nurses with Interpretive Statements and the AALNC Code of Ethics as ethical guides.
- Excess insurance coverage: This type of insurance policy is designed to provide coverage when expenses or damages reach a specific amount, normally covered by "umbrella coverage." This type of coverage may require the insured obtain an additional carrier.
- Exclusions: These are services or conditions listed within a policy that are not covered by the carrier.
- Exclusive jurisdiction: This type of jurisdiction limits a court to one form of legal action, or grants that only one court has the authority to rule on a specific type of action.
- Exhaust administrative remedies: This remedy requires that a plaintiff proceed with all available options prior to requesting judicial review.
- Ex-parte communications: This type of communication is a one-sided effort that appears to try to influence an official at a trial or hearing.
- Fact witness: In a lawsuit, this individual has information regarding the event in question, but is not a named defendant.
- Federal question jurisdiction: This jurisdiction grants authority to federal courts to resolve claims pertaining to federal law or Constitutional matters.
- Field case management: This type of case management involves personal contact with a client in a particular setting, such as a home, workplace, hospital, or physician's office.
- Foreseeability: The assumption that injuries sustained were foreseeable, or should have been foreseeable, based upon a substandard care practice of a health care provider.
- Frivolous claim: This type of claim is determined to have no basis in fact or in law.
- General acceptance test: This is the test for determining whether expert testimony is admissible based upon accepted standards.
- Guardian: The guardian is appointed by a judge to provide for the care and management of the assets and rights of another individual when the other individual is adjudged unable to do so as a result of defect of age, understanding, or self-control.

Copyright © Mometrix Media. You have been licensed one copy of this document for personal use only. Any other reproduction or redistribution is strictly prohibited. All rights reserved.

- Guardianship: A proceeding wherein a judge appoints a person to provide care for another individual who is under 18 years of age and/or to handle the estate of another individual.

- HCFA: This organization is known the Center for Medicare and Medicaid Services, but was previously the Health Care Finance Administration. The organization participated in nursing home regulation.

- HCPCS: This is the HCFA Common Procedural Coding System. Health care providers and suppliers utilize this uniform system to report services, procedures, and supplies.

- Headnotes: Headnotes comprise the numbered paragraphs of a court opinion. These paragraphs summarize relevant facts and laws.

- Hired gun: When referred to in legal terms, this individual is represented as a person who will provide sought after testimony in exchange for a fee.

- HMO: This refers to a Health Maintenance Organization. The health insurance organization enrolls members who can then obtain medical services from health care providers who also participate in the organization.

- ICD-9CM: This is the International Classification of Diseases and Clinical Modification. Medicare Part B requires the this three-digit code for disease reference, along with a one to two decimal point number for specificity.

- ID Code: This coding is utilized for identification of individual users. The code is issued by vendors for this purpose.

- IDEX: This organization specializes in recovering expert testimony on behalf of the defense bar.

- IDT: This is the Interdisciplinary Team. The team is made up of nurses, physicians, and therapists.

- Impeachment: When calling into question the credibility of a witness through presentation of information contrary to the testimony, the attorney is impeaching the witness.

- In camera: In law, this refers to a proceeding in a judge's private room

- In vitro study: Meaning "in glass," this type of study refers to a biologic or biochemical process outside a living organism.

- In vivo study: Meaning "in life," this type of study refers to a biologic or biochemical process in a living organism.

Copyright © Mometrix Media. You have been licensed one copy of this document for personal use only. Any other reproduction or redistribution is strictly prohibited. All rights reserved.

- Independent contractor: Relative to a LNC, this consultant is retained independently to provide consultation or expert testimony, and is not an employee of the retaining party.

- Inherent risk: A medical risk associated with a procedure or treatment that is present and conjoined with the treatment.

- Intellectual property: This property encompasses copyright, trademark, and patented materials.

- Intensity of service/severity of illness: This refers to the level of a patient's condition and the medical services required by him/her. This is also known as IS/SI.

- IPA: This is the Individual Practice Association. The association allows physicians to contract with particular plans. The services are then provided by the physician at an agreed-upon amount on a fee-for-service approach.

- IRB: This is the Institutional Review Board, comprising the committee involved in review of clinical studies. The protocols, informed consent documentation, and pertinent materials are evaluated to protect study subjects.

- Judgment notwithstanding the verdict: This is also known as "judgment non obstante verdicto" or JNOV, and pertains to a court's ruling overturning a jury decision when the judge feels the decision is not supported by the evidence.

- Judicial notice: Utilized as an evidentiary function, this notice grants evidence into admission without proof when quickly confirmed.

- Jury instructions: These instructions are given to the jury by the judge to serve as guidelines for deliberation of a verdict.

- Justice: Ethically, this doctrine dictates a duty to treat all persons fairly. With distributive justice, treatment is done as fairly as possible; in health care, this may be based upon the need of one individual being greater than the need of another.

- Kantianism: Under this viewpoint, the outcome of an action does not dictate whether it was right or wrong; right or wrong depends upon whether the action supported a principle.

- Learned treatises: Normally in the realm of textbooks, this type of document provides standards, methods, and principles related to care.

- Liberty interest: Federal and state constitution due process clauses protect this type of interest.

Copyright © Mometrix Media. You have been licensed one copy of this document for personal use only. Any other reproduction or redistribution is strictly prohibited. All rights reserved.

- Lien: An individual's or entity's claim against the asset of another individual or entity.
- Life-sustaining medical treatment: This type of treatment prevents a person's body from being legally dead by continuing the life functions.
- Limits: This represents the amount actually covered pursuant to an insurance policy.
- Loss control: This refers to an attempt to reduce losses in a cost-effective fashion by utilizing specific approaches.
- Material risk: When involved with treatment or medical care, this is the risk that might influence a patient's decision to consent to such treatment if he/she is informed regarding the same.
- MCO: This refers to a Managed Care Organization. MCOs include PPOs, HMOs, or EPOs. MCOs attempt to contain health care costs through various methods (e.g., network care, case management).
- MDS: This is the Minimum Data Set. The national medium is utilized to evaluate resident needs and establish reimbursement.
- Memorandum of law: This writing completely documents research and analysis of the legal basis of a specific point of law.
- Memorandum opinion: This court opinion is a ruling that does not detail the basis of the decision. This is normally a short document, since it does not elaborate.
- Middle range theory: Unlike a specific theory, a middle range can be somewhat limited in range, less abstract, and mirror practice.
- Morality: The common social viewpoints of right and wrong based upon how people live within a society and the values they hold.
- Motion for new trial: This pleading is filed by an attorney in a cause of action and asks that the court grant a new trial because of a prejudicial ruling.
- Motion in limine: This document is prepared for the pretrial. The document asks for issuance of an interlocutory order to restrain the opposition from presenting evidence the court has not confirmed is admissible.
- NANDA: This refers to the North American Nursing Diagnosis Association. The association participates in development and promotion of nursing diagnosis and its uses.
- NCQA: This refers to the National Committee for Quality Assurance. The NCQA is non-profit and independent organized to review clinical outcomes, contract

Copyright © Mometrix Media. You have been licensed one copy of this document for personal use only.
Any other reproduction or redistribution is strictly prohibited. All rights reserved.

practices, and surveys of its members. The review is designed to evaluate health care coverage of insurers and managed care organizations.

- NEC: This refers to information Not Elsewhere Classifiable, in that there is not a separate more distinct listing for a condition noted. The classification is used in Volume 2 of the ICD-9.
- NIC: This refers to the Nursing Interventions Classification. This system provides for placement of interventions into taxonomy.
- NOC: This refers to the Nursing Outcomes Classification. This system provides for placement of outcomes in a taxonomy.
- Nolo contendere: This is a form of plea wherein the accused party will not defend the allegations and will consent to punishment in the event of a guilty verdict.
- NOS: This refers to information Not Otherwise Specified, in that information cannot be assigned to a more distinct code based upon the information available. The classification is used in Volume 1 of the ICD-9.
- Notice of intent: The notice by a claimant to a health care provider or facility that the claimant has filed litigation against the provider or facility.
- OBRA: This refers to the Omnibus Budget Reconciliation Act of 1987. The Act modified nursing home standards of care through designation of minimum standards.
- Ombudsman: An ombudsman's responsibility is to represent citizens before government; this person is an official or semi-official with whom individuals may file government grievances.
- Opening statements: Each attorney's statements of the parties' intended proofs directed to the jury prior to admission of evidence.
- Original jurisdiction: This jurisdiction grants a court the authority to make the first ruling relative to law and facts in an action.
- Paradigm: The value and belief models shared by a profession's members.
- Paternalism: This ethical viewpoint extends beyond beneficence. With this point of view, the professional health care provider is considered to understand the best interest of the patient more appropriately than does the patient. To that end, the health care provider may act on behalf of the patient even when the patient disagrees.
- Pathognomic: This refers to anything representative of or exhibiting disease.
- Per curium: This term refers to an opinion handed down by an entire court.

Copyright © Mometrix Media. You have been licensed one copy of this document for personal use only. Any other reproduction or redistribution is strictly prohibited. All rights reserved.

- Persistent vegetative state: In this medical state, the patient is not able to voluntarily or purposefully act. The state involves continuing conscious impairment, when the patient reflexively responds only to painful stimuli.
- Pied Piper cases: This type of case involves vendors and similar individuals whose main business involves children and who have a duty to protect the safety of those who are unable to perceive danger.
- Pleadings: These documents encompass the written description of the allegations and defenses to the claim.
- PMPM: This represents per member per month, a formula designed to calculate the average utilization and cost for each plan member.
- Pocket parts: These documents are updates inserted in the back of a legal book or publication. The researcher should refer to these documents when researching case law to be sure no update relative to the particular case reviewed has been entered.
- PPO: This refers to a Preferred Provider Organization. This organization's plan members can receive benefits at a discount if the members use health care providers who contract with the plan.
- PPS: This is a Prospective Payment System. The system refers to payment based upon historical data relative to a variety of cases and contrasts in region.
- Prayer for relief: This paragraph(s) concludes the complaint and sets for the damages or remedies the plaintiff requests. This prayer is sometimes referred to as the ad damnum or Wherefore Clause.
- Preamble: This paragraph(s) appears at the beginning of a legal document and describes the purpose of the document.
- Pre-trial conference: This conference is held before a judge wherein all attorneys for parties to the action are present. At the hearing, the attorneys concur on certain issues to expedite trial procedure.
- Pretrial order: This written court order sets forth the process to be followed for orderly progression of a trial.
- Primary law: This is the type of law set forth by governmental bodies (legislatures, courts, or administrative agencies); basically, this is the "letter of the law."
- Principal investigator: This individual is also referred to as a PI. In health care, this individual is normally a physician qualified to handle research study trial conduct.

Copyright © Mometrix Media. You have been licensed one copy of this document for personal use only. Any other reproduction or redistribution is strictly prohibited. All rights reserved.

- Probate Court: This is the judiciary division of a county's superior court that handles probate matters such as decedent estates, guardianships, and conservatorships.
- Procedural law: These laws encompass the procedures that must occur to maintain rights and compel duties.
- Profit and loss: This represents the gain or loss as a result of goods bought or sold, or the gain or loss as a result of a business enterprise. In accounting practices, the gain is placed on the creditor's side and the loss is placed on the debtor's side.
- Proof chart: This provides a system that labels each fact to be proven and evidence to be presented in support.
- Properties of the nursing process: In the nursing process, these properties include purposeful, systematic, dynamic, interactive, and flexible.
- Provider: This refers to the party that supplies goods or services to another party (referred to as the beneficiary).
- Proximate cause: This legal concept places a limit upon the liability for the outcome of an individual's wrongful action.
- Quasi contract: This type of contract is designed to negate unjust enrichment and is implied in law.
- Question of fact: These facts involve the issues between parties to an action that caused the legal conflict.
- Question of law: These questions encompass the legal issues occurring during resolution of a cause of action.
- RAI: This refers to the Resident Assessment Instrument. This instrument is comprised of the MDS, RAPS, and care plan.
- RAP: This refers to the Resident Assessment Protocol. This protocol is utilized to designate issues identified as a result of MDS usage.
- Redaction: When identifying information is removed from a record, the data is redacted.
- Refereed journal: This refers to a professional journal publishing information only after complete and detailed evaluation by an author's counterparts.
- Relevant: A showing that leads to proof of a material fact.
- Res gestae: This encompasses remarks immediately prior to, during, or following an occurrence that results in a cause of action.

Copyright © Mometrix Media. You have been licensed one copy of this document for personal use only. Any other reproduction or redistribution is strictly prohibited. All rights reserved.

- Restatement (Third) Tort Products Liability Section 6: This statement communicates that a prescription drug or medical device is considered unsafe as a result of defective design based upon the fact that a reasonable health care provider would not prescribe the drug or device because the foreseeable therapeutic advantages do not outweigh the known foreseeable risks.
- Retainer: This represents monies paid in advance for legal services; these monies are held in trust pending performance of the services.
- Reversed: This action overturns the verdict or ruling of a lower court.
- RUG: This refers to the Resource Utilization Group. Under this federally mandated classification, residents are organized into one of 44 payment groupings.
- RVS: This refers to the Relative Value System. This system provides that a service be assigned a value multiplied by a cost factor.
- SART: This refers to the Sexual Response Team.
- Scheduling conference: A conference at which the judge and all attorneys concur on a timeline for progression of an action.
- Service of process: This involves the delivery of documentation in a legal action (e.g., summons and complaint) to a certain party. Service must be pursuant to the legal requirements of the court rules.
- Settlement brochure: A document prepared by plaintiff's attorney that sets forth the facts, liability, evidence, and authority to prove the plaintiff's case.
- Shepard's Citations: This system is designed to verify case law and is widely used by attorneys and courts.
- Shepardizing: Shepardizing involves the verification of law utilizing Shepard's Citations.
- Sine qua non: This means "essential prerequisite."
- Special purpose deposition summary: This document is prepared to contain specific testimony or testimony that pertains to additional research or documentation.
- Specific performance: This written order issued by a court requires that a party complete performance of a contract involving transfer of unique property.
- Steering committee: This committee is appointed by the judge in class action suits. The committee consists of attorneys and parties to the action who execute duties pursuant to court and lead counsel request.

Copyright © Mometrix Media. You have been licensed one copy of this document for personal use only. Any other reproduction or redistribution is strictly prohibited. All rights reserved.

- Sub rosa: A form of investigation done on behalf of the defendant; a private investigator's approach to investigation which involves videotape surveillance of a claimant.
- Subcontract: An express or implied contractual agreement entered into between a party on an original contract and a third party.
- Subcontractor: An individual or entity that enters into an express or implied contractual agreement with a person or entity already contracted for performance of a specific act; the subcontractor agrees to perform the act of the principal under the original contract.
- Subject matter jurisdiction: This jurisdiction allows a court to rule based upon the type of dispute before the court.
- Subpoena duces tecum: This document is a court order that requires an individual or representative to appear and present documents for inspection or copying.
- Subpoena: This document is a court order that requires an individual to appear for testimony.
- Substituted service: The delivery of documentation in a legal action that is accomplished by means other than through personal service to the party named in the document, normally through delivery to an individual appointed by an agent or to an agent pursuant to law.
- Summary judgment: This written order issued by a court gets rid of part or all of a civil action prior to court proceedings.
- Synopsis: This document briefly describes the facts and questions of law. The synopsis prefaces a court opinion.
- Technical nurse consultant: A nurse who possesses the skills and expertise necessary for computerized presentations in legal actions.
- Telephonic case management: This type of management involves organization of services utilizing telephone contact only.
- Tickler system: This system is utilized to note essential dates and deadlines. By utilizing this system, deadlines and issues that must be addressed are not missed.
- Topical deposition summary: This document is prepared to contain information relative to testimony on specific subjects.
- Trial brief: This pleading is prepared by an attorney for presentation to the court and is designed to outline the parties' legal and factual issues to be put before the court at the time of trial.

Copyright © Mometrix Media. You have been licensed one copy of this document for personal use only. Any other reproduction or redistribution is strictly prohibited. All rights reserved.

- Trial de novo: This refers to a new trial.
- Truncation: A system utilized to located words sharing a root or stem.
- U & C: This refers to Usual and Customary charges, a specified fee determined by health care charges consistent with the average rate for like services in a particular geographic region.
- UB-92: This refers to the Universal Bill 1992 form. Hospital-based health care providers utilize this form for billing for services rendered.
- URC: This refers to usual, reasonable, and customary, a system designed for determination of benefits. With this system, provider charges are compared to the charges of other providers in identical areas and specialties.
- Utilitarianism: The viewpoint that dictates actions are right if the majority benefit in a given circumstance.
- Venue: This grants that in litigation, the lawsuit is filed in the most advantageous location for trial occurrence.
- Voir dire: This is questioning that occurs during jury selection prior to trial. The questions are designed to ensure that a potential jury is not biased or prejudiced.
- Wrongful death: An action brought on behalf of a decedent's beneficiaries alleging the legal theory that the death was caused by the deliberate or negligent act of the defendant.
- Wrongful life: A medical malpractice claim filed on behalf of a child which alleges he/she would not have been born if not for negligent advice or treatment on behalf of the child's parents.

Copyright © Mometrix Media. You have been licensed one copy of this document for personal use only. Any other reproduction or redistribution is strictly prohibited. All rights reserved.

Risk Management

Risk

Risk is the potential that an individual may suffer harm or loss. To manage risk, health care facilities may purchase insurance to cover liability or the facility may attempt to reduce or prevent loss. Thus, many institutions have developed risk management programs. These programs concentrate on the risks involved with patients in the facility and the possibility they may suffer harm. When a patient suffers an injury and the health care facility is required to compensate the patient, the associated expenses are a loss to the institution. Thus, the risk management program is designed to develop a plan that will not only identify and analyze risks, but reduce and monitor those risks. Primarily, risk management is designed to reduce the occurrence of negative incidents and the liability and financial loss that can result from malpractice and other civil claims.

Loss control and transfer of risk

Two areas of risk control include loss control and transfer of risk. Loss control involves monitoring the incidence of loss. An example of monitoring might be using side rails on beds. Loss control also deals with reducing the intensity of the loss. With this type of loss control, the facility's representative may work with the patient and family immediately after an incident occurs in an attempt to decrease the possibility of a claim. Transfer of risk involves an agreement holding another party responsible for payment for a loss. To accomplish transfer of risk, a "hold harmless" clause is included in the agreement. In this way, one party agrees to hold the other party "harmless" from liability in the event of injury. Additionally, a subrogation clause in the contract may provide that one party agrees to substitute in the place of another party in the event a claim is filed.

Loss prevention and the techniques utilized to reduce claims

Loss prevention is designed to reduce the occurrence of injury, as well as the financial loss sustained by health care institutions. Loss prevention is normally utilized to prevent loss, rather than insure against loss. To that end, health care institutions should attempt to meet

Copyright © Mometrix Media. You have been licensed one copy of this document for personal use only. Any other reproduction or redistribution is strictly prohibited. All rights reserved.

all needs of a patient to grant him/her some control over his/her health care and the ability to manage health issues. Also, the facility's health care providers should do all possible to maintain the patient's sense of dignity while working with the patient. Health care facilities do not always meet these needs, especially in the areas of patient privacy and respect of the patient's dignity. Studies demonstrate that most injured patients do not institute malpractice claims, and many that do have not actually sustained an injury. Therefore, nurses must develop effective communication skills.

Risk financing

Risk financing is a form of transferring risk. This type of financing deals with insurance contracts. The contract states that for a premium paid, a party will compensate the party paying the premium if the event of a loss in a specific area of risk. The institution purchases financing through risk retention or an insurance policy. Risk retention involves an institution's plan to fund all risks internally. The funding is normally through company assets or proceeds. The institution may choose to fund the risk partially through insurance and risk retention. When an organization maintains a specific risk retention fund, self-insurance is practiced. If the organization assumes the risk without a specific fund to pay claims, the institution is "going bare."

Nurse's challenges relative to quality patient care

The nurse must meet the demands of coordinating managed care in a cost-effective manner with the demands of standards of care. The nurse, though, is mainly a patient advocate and a patient caregiver, and his/her focus must be in these roles. If the nurse is unable to retain this focus, he/she will add to the current loss of patient and quality care being suffered in the health care environment. In doing so, the nurse may increase his/her liability risk. The nurse can alleviate some of the pressure of quality care loss through involvement in committees and organizations designed to reinforce patient care.

Nurse's roles

Nurses possess the skills granting them the chance to identify possible areas of risk. Nurses are also able to identify circumstances that may cause harm to patients. Nurses are able to contribute to programs developed to decrease nurse liability, through utilizing their

Copyright © Mometrix Media. You have been licensed one copy of this document for personal use only. Any other reproduction or redistribution is strictly prohibited. All rights reserved.

knowledge and experience. Nurses also possess research and administrative abilities, which can be utilized to assemble relevant information that can be used for policies and procedures that will reduce risks. Nurses are also able to identify high-risk practice areas and offer input to reduce the risk. Safety issues are within the special knowledge of nurses as well. Nurses can review incident reports and patient care programs to locate safety issues.

Compliance with risk management procedures

When health care providers comply with the policies and procedures developed by the risk management team of a health care facility, several benefits can be realized. Compliance can result in loss prevention, loss reduction involving legal actions, and loss reduction in expenses relative to regulatory requirements. Also, the procedures developed help to provide structure in the facility's operation. The employees receive guidance in the workplace, which can translate to positive standards of care. A safe work and patient environment can result from compliance with policies. Patients can benefit from reduction in occurrences that may result in injury. If the policies are developed in a manner to meet statutory and regulatory mandates, the institution's licensing and accreditation may be positively affected.

Noncompliance with risk management procedures

The policies and procedures developed for an institution act to identify the facilities' standards. If health care providers fail to meet the policies and procedures developed, the institution may be subject to liability and loss of professional standing. The liability claims may be instituted by employees, contractors providing services, the public, or patients. Also, noncompliance can lead to adverse actions by regulators, accreditors, and reimbursers. An adverse action can take the form of loss of a health care provider's license or reimbursement issues that can cause financial losses. Additional costs may be sustained to defend legal actions brought by individuals or regulatory agencies.

Utilization review process

The utilization review (UR) process provides for evaluation of appropriate, quality, and necessary medical services. Trained specialists in specific disciplines conduct this review

Copyright © Mometrix Media. You have been licensed one copy of this document for personal use only. Any other reproduction or redistribution is strictly prohibited. All rights reserved.

of recommended services. Normally, personnel other than physicians perform the evaluation to determine whether the treatment recommended is necessary. If the personnel determine the treatment is not medically necessary, they may refer the matter to a physician for further review. The health care provider is notified if the physician also believes the treatment is not necessary. The health care provider can appeal the decision. Specific areas considered in the event of an appeal include consultation, medical records, independent medical examinations, and review by the UR board.

Peer review process and immunity

Peer review is designed to monitor and evaluate an organization's health care provider's patient care. The Health Care Financing Administration (HCFA) provides peer review services to determine medical necessity, reasonableness, and appropriate standards of care. The review may include assessment of individual performance. A negative review relative to an individual's practices can result in restrictions or termination. The National Practitioner Data Bank, National Council of State Boards of Nursing Data Bank, or other organizations may be notified of the negative report. If an individual participates in the peer review process, he/she may be granted "immunity" from a civil lawsuit. Since the process is designed to achieve quality improvement, patient care improvement, and morbidity and mortality rate reduction, many states recognize immunity.

Quality assurance

Quality assurance programs attempt to provide standards of care, measure patient care relative to standards set, review charts, interview patient health care providers, and oversee patient care. The programs also allow for recommendations to improve areas of concern. The care provided by nursing staff should be evaluated relative to competence, subject matter, resources, and end results. The programs assist in locating areas of patient care that can be improved, liability reduction, and forwarding nursing goals. Nurses should participate in quality assurance programs to ensure quality care for their patients. Liability claims can be numerous in the medical arena, and nurses can protect themselves from claims by monitoring standards of care. The programs grant nurses an opportunity to identify and solve issues in their specific environment. After identifying issues, nurses are granted the chance to implement plans in their health care environment.

Copyright © Mometrix Media. You have been licensed one copy of this document for personal use only. Any other reproduction or redistribution is strictly prohibited. All rights reserved.

Identify risk

Risk can be identified either formally or informally. When identifying risk in an informal manner, the source may be the "grapevine" or media reports. Formally, the source may be a report or committee meeting. The source may also be a patient or family member formal complaint or review of a facility survey the patient or family may have completed. Additionally, the facility may receive a complaint from a health care provider. Reviews performed by administrative agencies (e.g., National Committee on Performance Improvement) will also identify risk areas, as well an investigation performed by an agency such as OSHA. The risk management department may also review the facility's policies. Obviously, a summons and complaint initiating litigation is formal risk identification.

Types of risks that should be reported

Anesthesia-related injury, birth-related injury, and iatrogenic injury should be formally reported. Foreign body retention and any medication mistake should be reported. Unexpected incidents, such as death, neurological or sensory issues, respiratory or cardiopulmonary arrest (when resuscitation is not successful), and body-system failure, need to be reported to the risk management department. The nurse should report incidents that occur within the hospital that reduce the daily activities of a patient or staff member, result in a drug-drug and food-drug reactions (allergic in nature or otherwise), or allege sexual assault. Other incidents to report include suicides, burns from medical devices or other sources, or wrong-site surgery. Also, a patient leaving against medical advice or leaving without the knowledge of staff or health care providers should be reported.

Process of risk assessment consultation

The LNC can perform risk assessments in risk management, which may include clinical or specialty area assessments. The assessments may also be that of property and casualty or directors' and officers' risks. The LNC can develop expertise in any of these areas. When a clinical assessment is performed, an on-site visit normally occurs. This type of assessment usually involves high risk, large volume areas and those tending toward problems. The clinical process involves personal interviews with pertinent personnel or staff, review of records and charts, committee records (e.g., minutes) that address risk areas, and a walk-

Copyright © Mometrix Media. You have been licensed one copy of this document for personal use only. Any other reproduction or redistribution is strictly prohibited. All rights reserved.

through of the facility's problematic area. The assessment may include the entire facility or may involve a specific area of the institution, such as a particular department.

Copyright © Mometrix Media. You have been licensed one copy of this document for personal use only. Any other reproduction or redistribution is strictly prohibited. All rights reserved.

Law

Nurse practice acts

Because nursing know requires additional education, technical skills, and business expertise, nurse practice acts have been passed by various state legislatures. These acts encompass statutes designed to define and regulate the area of nursing. The acts not only define nursing, but also set standards for nurses. Each state enacts its own nurse practice acts, although most tend to utilize the American Nurses Association or National Council of State Boards of Nursing regulations. By setting standards, the acts help to protect patients and establish a nursing standard of care. Criminal prosecution, disciplinary action, or medical malpractice liability can result from violation of the acts.

Law

The behavior and interaction of people in a society is governed by specific rules and regulations. Those rules and regulations are known as laws. The purpose of laws is to resolve discord without violence, resulting in an ordered society. Laws also set forth individuals' duties and safeguard citizen health, safety, and welfare. Laws generally change to work with the current society, although some have been in effect almost constantly. Federal and state governments may enact and implement laws pursuant to the United States Constitution. The federal government maintains certain powers granted by the Constitution. State governments are entitled to powers not specifically granted to the federal government in the document. Article 1, Section 8, of the Constitution covers health care involvement relative to the federal government. This Article deals with general welfare and interstate commerce. Normally, either the state or federal government maintains authority to monitor health care through police power, which grants citizen protection of health, safety, and welfare.

Four sources of law in the United States
- Constitutional law: These laws offer fundamental principles relative to governmental power and organization. The Bill of Rights protects personal liberties and encompasses the basic health care and nursing practice area of the Constitution.

Copyright © Mometrix Media. You have been licensed one copy of this document for personal use only. Any other reproduction or redistribution is strictly prohibited. All rights reserved.

- Statutory law: These laws encompass federal, state, and local statutes, or formal written laws, enacted through legislation. The United States Code (U.S.C.) is the publication offering federal statutes. Several publications offer state statutes (e.g., Revised Codes Annotated).

- Administrative law: Administrative agencies develop administrative laws under the scope of the executive branch. The administrative agency retains authority to maintain enacted regulations. Health care providers are subject to responsibilities pursuant to the administrative law system.

- Common law: This type of law may have its origins in either English common law or in written civil code. Court decisions establish common laws when no existing statute or regulation is available to resolve an issue.

Emergency Medical Treatment and Active Labor Act

The Emergency Medical Treatment and Active Labor Act (EMTALA) was passed in 1986. The Act bans Medicare-participating emergency facilities from refusing service to patients without insurance or who are unable to pay. A facility is required to conduct a sufficient medical screening exam within the boundaries of its ability. Also, the Act requires that a patient can be transferred after certain conditions have occurred, including the medical screening, stabilization, and the patient has been cleared by the receiving facility. Pursuant to the Act, a patient is considered stabilized when the facility can insure no material deterioration will result from or during transfer. Violation of EMTALA guidelines can result in penalties of up to $50,000 per occurrence if a facility has more than 100 beds and up to $25,000 per occurrence with less than 100 beds.

Antitrust Laws and Trade Restrictions

Pursuant to federal and state antitrust laws, anticompetitive actions (e.g., monopolies or boycotts) are prohibited when commerce or trade may be hampered. Nurses may be affected by antitrust laws if employed in expanded roles. The Sherman Antitrust Act of 1890 provides that the government has the authority to commence criminal prosecution against an individual who develops a monopoly or sustains restrictive business agreements. The Clayton Act of 1914, as amended by the Robinson-Patman Act, also makes certain practices that involve monopolies illegal. This Act was adopted to supplement the

Copyright © Mometrix Media. You have been licensed one copy of this document for personal use only. Any other reproduction or redistribution is strictly prohibited. All rights reserved.

Sherman Antitrust Act. The Clayton Act confirms the rights of union pickets, boycotts, or strikes and provides for labor dispute resolution. The Federal Trade Commission Act of 1914 provides that "unfair methods of competition" are illegal. Enforcement of antitrust laws and the ability to issue cease and desist orders are included in the Commission's responsibilities. States also enact laws and restrictions to protect the public health (e.g.., nurse practice acts). Some state laws and restrictions involve AIDS, abuse, and Good Samaritan laws.

Administrative Agencies

Department of Health and Human Services
Department of Health and Human Services: The federal government executive branch maintains control of the DHHS. This department maintains the main source of rules for health care. The DHHS has five operating divisions to enforce regulations.

Federal Council on Aging
The President receives advice and assistance relative to the needs of the elderly from the FCOA.

National Institute on Aging
The NIA operates under the arm of the National Institutes of Health. The NIA conducts and supports research and training involved in the care of diseases of elderly Americans.

State Boards of Nursing
These state boards are state administrative agencies designed to develop and enforce nursing practice regulations.

Divisions of the Department of Health and Human Services

The divisions of the DHHS are the Health Care Financing Administration, Office of Human Development Services, Family Support Administration, Public Health Service, and Social Security Administration. The Health Care Financing Administration retains responsibility for Medicare and Medicaid programs and their quality assurance, Medicare policy and procedure development and implementation, and grants for indigent medical services through Medicaid. The Public Health Service (PHS) is designed to safeguard mental and

Copyright © Mometrix Media. You have been licensed one copy of this document for personal use only. Any other reproduction or redistribution is strictly prohibited. All rights reserved.

physical health by execution of laws and policies, including research, education, and expertise of all health facilities. The PHS also controls the Food and Drug Administration (FDA) and the National Institutes of Health. The Social Security Administration retains responsibility for the social insurance program and retirement income, including disability and death benefits. This division's funding source is employer and employee contributions. The DHHS also maintains responsibility for the Supplemental Security Income program, Medicaid, Medicare, and the Older American Act programs.

State Boards of Nursing

State Boards of Nursing are maintains to regulate nursing practice and licensing. The administrative laws of the Boards are legally binding. The Boards' authority encompasses the reprimand, probation, suspension, or revocation of nursing licenses if allegations warrant such decisions. The Boards are overseen by the National Council of State Boards of Nursing. This non-profit organization oversees Boards in the 50 states, as well as several territories (e.g., District of Columbia, Guam, and Samoa). The Council allows the Boards to work together on issues of public safety, health, and welfare. The Council develops the NCLEX-PN and NCLEX-RN examinations, distributes nurse licensure data, conducts relevant research and policy evaluation, provides consistent practice regulations, and provides an area to share information. The nurse aide's competency evaluation program was formed by the Council.

Common law and the civil code

Common law, developed through court decisions that become law, is followed in 49 states and the federal courts. Common law varies from state to state, since state court decisions differ among each state. Civil code, on the other hand, is law authorized by legislature. Civil codes form an extensive organization of general regulations; common law is based upon individual case issues. Civil law originates from Roman law; common law originates from English law. With common law, court decisions become "stare decisis," or "to stand by things decided." Courts, therefore, may utilize previous court decisions to rule on a case before the court. This utilization of previous court decisions is known as "precedent." Ordinarily, courts will make decisions based upon prior law or decisions of higher courts. Malpractice issues are normally decided pursuant to common law.

Copyright © Mometrix Media. You have been licensed one copy of this document for personal use only. Any other reproduction or redistribution is strictly prohibited. All rights reserved.

Substantive law, procedural law, statute of limitations, and civil

Substantive law: This type of law defines the particular harm or obligation involved in litigation that results in trial. Substantive law plays a role upon filing a lawsuit.

Procedural law: This type of law defines the process that guides the violation of the individual or organizational right. This law provides rules to follow when bringing an action before the court. Procedural law also plays a role in lawsuits.

Statute of limitations: This type of law sets forth time limitations for a claimant to file a lawsuit. Statute of limitations falls under procedural law.

Civil law: This type of law encompasses individual and organizations rights and protections. A party may receive a monetary award as a result of litigation brought pursuant to civil law.

Contract law and tort law

Contract law encompasses agreements involving two or more parties. The agreements set forth responsibilities of all parties involved. The contractual agreement contains the offer, acceptance, and consideration given in exchange for the service set forth in the agreement (e.g., money). Both oral and written contracts are considered binding, although some types must be in written form to enforce. The responsibilities between the parties may be either implied or express. Employment agreements are the common form experienced by nurses. In this case, the written form of contract is best and easier to challenge and uphold. Tort law encompasses negligence and malpractice. Thus, nurses are more familiar with tort law, rather than civil law. Tort law involves unintentional tort and intentional tort.

Criminal law, misdemeanor, and felony.

Criminal law deals with crimes and the punishment imposed as a result of conviction. These laws are designed to protect the public. The written criminal statutes or codes define the laws. The plaintiff in a criminal prosecution is a governmental agency and the defendant is the person or entity violating the law. The health field does not normally experience criminal law violations. However, nurses can be subject to charges in the event

Copyright © Mometrix Media. You have been licensed one copy of this document for personal use only. Any other reproduction or redistribution is strictly prohibited. All rights reserved.

of life support withheld from newborns or terminally ill patients or for narcotic record alteration. In addition, nurses may provide testimony at criminal hearings if he/she has provided care for a victim. Misdemeanors involve violations of criminal law, but are normally thought of as lesser crimes. These violations normally involve fines or imprisonment as punishment. Felonies, however, are serious crimes and can carry severe punishment (e.g., fine, imprisonment, death sentence). Monetary awards are not granted in criminal proceedings; rather, the defendant is punished by loss of liberty or life.

Criminal process

Both federal and state criminal actions involve the same basic steps. First, the defendant is indicted pursuant to a document containing all allegations. Second, the defendant is subject to grand jury review to determine whether there is sufficient proof of a crime; this step is utilized regularly by federal courts, but only by some state courts. Third, the defendant is arraigned, at which time he/she enters a plea of guilty or not guilty, and the court sets bail. The defendant is released if the defendant makes bail, but taken into custody if unable to do so. Fourth, discovery proceeds to gather evidence on both sides of the proceeding. Fifth, pretrial motions are filed and heard by the court. The motions are designed to reduce trial time by resolving issues prior to commencement of trial. Last, the action proceeds to trial, where witness testimony is heard and evidence is presented. The jury will make a decision of guilty or not guilty at the conclusion of testimony and evidence presentation. The defendant will be sentenced if found guilty and may appeal the decision if he/she wishes to do so.

Fraud

When a party intentionally misrepresents a statement he/she knows to be false, while aware that the misrepresentation may provide an illegal benefit to his/herself or another individual, fraud is perpetrated. Normally, when health care fraud occurs, Medicare is involved. The types of fraud may include kickbacks, billing for non-rendered care or treatment (e.g., visits that did not occur), misrepresentation of a diagnosis for payment, falsifying documents, unbundling charges, waiver of deductibles or co-payments, billing for testing or treatment that is determined unnecessary, and inflated billings. A nurse who becomes aware of Medicaid fraud should notify the Medicaid and Medicare hotline established by the Office of the Inspector General (1-800-HHS-TIPS).

Copyright © Mometrix Media. You have been licensed one copy of this document for personal use only. Any other reproduction or redistribution is strictly prohibited. All rights reserved.

Jurisdiction

Each court maintains authority to make a decision in legal matters; this authority is known as jurisdiction. When a plaintiff files a complaint, the court accepts the action based upon whether or not it has jurisdiction. Federal and state constitutions and statutes determine the authority of each court to hear a case. Federal issues and disagreements between residents of different states fall within federal court jurisdiction. Some courts have overall jurisdictions to decide cases, while other courts may have specific or specialized jurisdiction (e.g., traffic courts, probate courts). A party bringing an action may decide which court will hear and decide his/her case if more than one court (e.g., a state and a federal court) has jurisdiction.

Court system

The United States has established the federal court system and the state court system. Article III, Section 11, of the United States Constitution grants judicial power in the United States Supreme Court, and Congress has granted some authority in lesser federal courts. Each state and the federal court system maintain trial courts, appellate courts, and a Court of Appeals or Supreme Court (the highest appellate court). Once a party appeals an action through the levels of the state court system, he/she/it may attempt an appeal to the United States Supreme Court. The US Supreme Court does not hear most cases appealed to it. The appeal is attempted through a writ of certiorari requesting the Supreme Court hear the case, and the Court then grants or denies the appeal. Likewise, under the federal system, a party can try to appeal circuit court decisions to the United States Supreme Court.

Trial courts

The trial court is the first court in the legal system. A plaintiff files the complaint or petition in the local, state, or district court, or in the United States federal court to request a remedy for damages. The defendant then answers the complaint. The discovery process commences in preparation for trial or alternative dispute resolution. The trial decision may be rendered by a jury or judge, dependent upon the laws governing the specific court system. The proceedings are monitored by the judge, who also determines questions of law. The judge or jury renders a verdict. The party against whom the verdict is rendered

Copyright © Mometrix Media. You have been licensed one copy of this document for personal use only. Any other reproduction or redistribution is strictly prohibited. All rights reserved.

may appeal the decision. A jury or judge decides the outcome of medical malpractice actions based upon the facts and whether standards of care were breached and injury to plaintiff resulted from such breach.

Appellate courts

While the trial court is the first step in the legal system, the appellate courts (either state appellate courts or the United States Court of Appeals) have the power to review and amend state or federal trial court decisions. The case appealed, however, must be within the appellate court's jurisdiction and authority. The federal system maintains 12 circuit courts, each circuit comprising 3 to 9 states. Unlike trial courts, no testimony or witnesses are heard, and no jury is present. The case is reviewed and decided strictly based upon the trial transcript and briefs presented by each party's attorney. The appellate court has the authority to affirm or reverse the lower court's decision, as well as remand the action back to the lower court along with instructions for proceeding after appeal. Appellate court decisions can be researched in "reporters."

Supreme courts

The appellate courts hear appeals from trial courts. The step beyond the appellate court is the supreme court. State supreme courts are normally the final appeal arena for state issues, unless a federal or constitutional issue is to be decided. All courts within the particular state are bound by rulings of the state supreme court. The United States Supreme Court is the final court to which a party may appeal a decision of a lower court. Also, the United States Supreme Court hears appeals on matters of constitutionally protected rights (e.g., freedom of speech). All state and federal courts throughout the United States are bound by the final ruling of the United States Supreme Court.

Plaintiff and defendant

The plaintiff is the individual or entity that brings a lawsuit in a state or federal court. The plaintiff alleges injury or damages and requests remedies in the form of a monetary or other award. The plaintiff may be the actual individual harmed or may be the legal guardian or next of kin of a deceased individual. The defendant is the individual or entity against whom the plaintiff brings the action. The defendant is the party claimed to have

Copyright © Mometrix Media. You have been licensed one copy of this document for personal use only. Any other reproduction or redistribution is strictly prohibited. All rights reserved.

caused plaintiff's injury or damages. A medical malpractice claim may name a nurse, physician, HMO, insurance company, health care facility, pharmaceutical company, medical device company, or any health care provider as a defendant.

Copyright © Mometrix Media. You have been licensed one copy of this document for personal use only. Any other reproduction or redistribution is strictly prohibited. All rights reserved.

Life Care Planning

Life care plan in catastrophic personal injury actions

The life care plan is designed to provide an estimate of care for a plaintiff with a catastrophic or permanent injury. This plan is essential to the plaintiff's remedies requested in the complaint. The plan includes a complete assessment of the plaintiff's needs over an extended period of time. The plan should relate to the plaintiff's disability after the injury or illness was sustained. Costs associated with any pre-existing illness are not part of the estimations. A life care plan is developed to set forth the needs of a particular individual and to encourage independence and well-being. The plan should also be objective and uniform throughout, as well as provide a lifelong, but adjustable, assessment and estimate. Finally, the plan should be comprehensive and information should have a multidisciplinary foundation.

Life care plan when assessing damages

The life care planner should educate all parties and the jury regarding the consequences of the plaintiff's injury upon his/her life. The planner should analyze the individual's medical, allied medical, and psychosocial requirements and be able to set forth an intelligible idea of the costs (both economic and non-economic) associated with the injury. The plaintiff's position can be strengthened by credible information that outlines his/her future requirements. In the event of trial, the jury will benefit from a well-written and documented life care plan. The plan will allow the jury to understand the plaintiff's monetary demand based upon future needs, as well as the types of care that will be required. The defendant's attorney may retain a planner to assist in cross-examination or to offer alternatives to the plaintiff's needs.

Requirements of a qualified life care planner

The most essential factor in choosing an expert life care planner is credibility. The planner's education, experience relative to the actual damages of the case, credentials, communication abilities, and professional expertise are factors to consider when retaining

Copyright © Mometrix Media. You have been licensed one copy of this document for personal use only. Any other reproduction or redistribution is strictly prohibited. All rights reserved.

the life care planner. Also, the planner should possess rehabilitation expertise, with meaningful hand-on experience. Case management experience is essential, including coordinating services similar to those proposed for plaintiff. The planner should be able to locate health care providers and vendors with the ability to provide for plaintiff's needs. The plaintiff's needs, age, and diagnosis should also be considered when choosing a life care planner; one that has professional experience with similar individuals is necessary. The life care planner's credentials should be impeccable, including continuing education relative to current practices.

Required Certifications

The various specialty certifications a rehabilitation nurse might have to aid in Certified Registered Rehabilitation Nurse (C.R.R.N.) – This certification assists with rehabilitation needs, especially when dealing with understanding and explaining intricate needs associated with severe injury. This certification is also helpful when a pre-existing condition is involved.

Certified Case Manager (C.C.M.) – This certification demonstrates multidisciplinary experience involved in organizing rehabilitation services.

Certified Rehabilitation Counselor (C.R.C.) or Certified Disability Management Specialist (C.D.M.S.) – This certification assists with assessment of restructuring the plaintiff's employment abilities.

Certified Life Care Planner (C.L.C.P.) – This certification demonstrates multidisciplinary experience relative to life care plan preparation.

Certified Nurse Life Care Planner (C.N.L.C.P.) – This certification demonstrates experience with life care plan preparation.

Steps required to complete a life care plan

First, the injured party's needs must be assessed and medical records reviewed. This assessment may include a meeting with the injured party, usually in his/her home environment. The primary caregiver should be present at the meeting. Second, the actual

Copyright © Mometrix Media. You have been licensed one copy of this document for personal use only. Any other reproduction or redistribution is strictly prohibited. All rights reserved.

needs must be determined in detail. The medical records and information from health care providers will assist in this determination. The determination should include the services as related to damages and possible changes that may occur. Third, costs must be determined; the planner utilizes today's dollars for costs. Normally, an economist is retained to evaluate the costs relative to inflation, interest rates, and economic impacts. Fourth, the report is formulated and written, if requested. Last, the life care plan may be reviewed, normally by the defendant's attorney to support the defense case.

Components of the life care plan

First, the life care planner should be sure a written report is needed, rather than just a verbal assessment. If a written report is requested, the planner should use care in preparing a detailed and clear outline of the party's injuries and the needs associated with the injuries. The plan will present justifiable and organized damages, while presenting the medical needs, family make-up and culture, values, and premorbid lifestyle of the injured party. Normally, the planner will start with a short summary of the party's past and present medical status and the impact the injury in question has had on the plaintiff. The planner must speak to all areas of the party's care. Future medical care estimations should include all health care provider costs and costs for testing and hospitalization. Medical devices and equipment must be considered when estimating costs as well, including replacement and maintenance. Any modifications to plaintiff's residence should be detailed. The estimated costs should be organized by procedure and the age of the claimant. A summary table is helpful when showing these costs.

Nurse life care planner's role

A defense attorney may retain a nurse life care planner to either review the plaintiff's life care plan or to prepare an independent life care plan with alternative assessments and estimations. The defense life care planner will review those issues set forth in the claimant's plan. The review will include the plan's suitability to the injury, whether it is pertinent to the damages alleged in the lawsuit, whether the costs are plausible, and the location of services available to plaintiff. The nurse life care planner should conduct a personal interview with the plaintiff, if possible.   The planner can be helpful relative to possible sources of pre-existing conditions related to the injuries relevant to the litigation. The planner should also research possible collateral sources of services for plaintiff. These

Copyright © Mometrix Media. You have been licensed one copy of this document for personal use only. Any other reproduction or redistribution is strictly prohibited. All rights reserved.

alternative sources may be admissible as evidence only under certain rules of evidence, but if admitted, can show the plaintiff will receive the necessary care even if not awarded damages.

Legal and ethical principles to be considered

The life care plan should represent a truthful illustration of the claimant's injuries and needs. The life care planner should provide a representation that educates the jury, court, and attorney regarding the plaintiff's condition. Thus, the plan should be impartial, whether prepared on behalf of the plaintiff or defendant. The life care planner should consider the plaintiff's quality of life. The services and care evaluated should help to re-establish plaintiff's lifestyle. The plan should also relate specifically to the plaintiff and his/her conditions. All funding sources and costs should be enumerated in detail, including collateral sources available. The planner should attempt to provide care in the plaintiff's local area. The life care planner should not consider liability, causation, or standard of care in the plan, since the plan is not developed for this purpose.

Deposition preparation

The life care planner should review all pertinent medical records prior to the deposition. The records should include those records gathered from the date of the report preparation to the date of the deposition. An update regarding plaintiff's condition should be obtained from the plaintiff or his/her caregiver; this applies to both plaintiff's and defendant's expert planner. The life care planner should also review the action with the attorney, since the deposition testimony will be similar to trial testimony. The life care planner should review all anticipated questions with the attorney prior to deposition to be properly prepared with relevant information. The opposing attorney will commence questioning at the deposition, and he/she will utilize the most time during the deposition. The retaining attorney will probably ask questions near the end of the deposition simply to clarify information. The planner's answers should be consistent, clear, and credible.

Trial testimony

The life care planner should review the all relevant records pertaining to plaintiff's damages. The planner should also update all records prior to trial. The planner may wish

Copyright © Mometrix Media. You have been licensed one copy of this document for personal use only. Any other reproduction or redistribution is strictly prohibited. All rights reserved.

to speak with health care providers, as well as plaintiff and his/her caregiver, to update plaintiff's condition. The life care planner should be knowledgeable about the life care plan and updated information to avoid referring to records during testimony. The life care planner may also wish to review his/her deposition transcript. Then, the life care planner should review the action with the retaining attorney, especially regarding possible cross-examination questioning. The life care planner should try to be present for as much trial testimony as possible. Since his/her testimony will likely occur near the end of the proceeding, it can be helpful to be aware of the testimony of other witnesses. When the planner is called to testify, credentials will be the likely initial subject. The planner must present him/herself as credible and knowledgeable to impress the jury. A nurse life care planner can refer to the state nurse practice acts to support expert testimony.

Copyright © Mometrix Media. You have been licensed one copy of this document for personal use only. Any other reproduction or redistribution is strictly prohibited. All rights reserved.

Criminal/Forensic

Criminal law and intent

Criminal acts are seldom connected to negligent actions. Also, criminal punishment does not normally involve monetary awards or damages. A criminal act must involve the elements of mens rea and actus reus (guilty intent and wrongful conduct). The LNC should be familiar with the specific statutes of the state in which the case is to be heard. Several levels of criminal intent exist. General intent involves an individual who participates in an everyday he/she should have known would result in criminal consequences, and the conviction results from the showing of the actual criminal act. An example of general intent is drug possession. Specific intent involves the act of knowingly participating in an activity that will result in a specific criminal consequence. An example of specific intent is breaking and entering.

Burden of proof in criminal actions

The prosecution maintains the burden of proof in all criminal actions. This requirements applies to both felony and misdemeanor cases. The defense counsel does not have any burden of proof in a criminal case. A person accused of a crime has the right to remain silent and decline testifying pursuant to the Fifth Amendment of the United States Constitution. The prosecutor must also prove guilt "beyond a reasonable doubt." Although the definition of "beyond a reasonable doubt" varies, it is normally accepted as being doubt based upon common sense and normal reason. Thus, the jury or judge must view the evidence as being credible, logical, and truthful.

"Not guilty" verdict and the right to a speedy trial

A not guilty verdict results from the prosecutor's failure to provide evidence of the criminal action beyond a reasonable doubt. Pursuant to the Fifth Amendment of the United States Constitution, an accused person cannot be subjected to a second trial, commonly referred as "double jeopardy." This provision also applies to the prosecutor's inability to bring charges for criminal acts that must utilize evidence relative to the same elements involved

Copyright © Mometrix Media. You have been licensed one copy of this document for personal use only.
Any other reproduction or redistribution is strictly prohibited. All rights reserved.

in the previous action. The Sixth Amendment grants that an accused person has the right to a speedy trial, the right to face his accuser, and proper legal representation at trial. If the defendant shows that the attorney representing him/her is incompetent and such incompetence will prejudice the defendant, a guilty verdict may be overturned if appealed. U.S. vs. Cronic and Strickland vs. Washington are used to apply the criteria of prejudice and competence.

Direct and indirect evidence

Testimonial, physical, and scientific evidence encompass the three types of evidence involved in criminal actions. The evidence can be presented as direct or indirect. If the evidence is direct, it demonstrates fact (e.g., an eye-witness). If the evidence is indirect, it is considered competent, but demonstrates a fact or element by relation only. Indirect evidence may be utilized when direct evidence is not available to establish a relationship. The LNC must review all medical evidence in criminal actions to determine whether the evidence is direct or indirect and how each piece may be utilized in trial.

Testimonial evidence

Testimony evidence is verbal evidence offered by witnesses and parties to the action. The verbal testimony may be from parties present during the criminal act, investigators after the act, and individuals who dispute the defendant's involvement in the act. As a result of Miranda vs. Arizona, the defendant's words may be used against him/her at trial, whether or not the defendant testifies. If the defendant's words are to be used by the prosecutor at trial, the defendant's statement must have been given freely, without undue influence. The defendant must also have been informed of his/her Miranda rights and that he/she fully understood those rights.

Physical evidence

All tangible objects offered as proof of a criminal act are considered physical evidence. Examples include guns, knives, or drugs. The Fourth Amendment of the United States Constitution protects individuals from unreasonable search and seizure. The prosecution must show that all physical evidence was gathered while protecting the defendant's search and seizure rights. Abandoned property is not protected, nor is evidence gathered when in

Copyright © Mometrix Media. You have been licensed one copy of this document for personal use only.
Any other reproduction or redistribution is strictly prohibited. All rights reserved.

view of a law enforcement officer. A search warrant must be obtained to gather evidence protected under the Fourth Amendment. The warrant can be issued only when the law enforcement officer shows probable cause showing that an offense is or may be perpetrated.

Scientific evidence

With scientific evidence, tangible items and technology join to prove or disprove guilt. Types of scientific testing include fingerprints, DNA, saliva, semen, and blood. The admissibility of evidence generally falls under the Federal Rules of Evidence, specifically Federal Rule of Evidence 702. In addition, Rule 702 controls admissibility of expert witness testimony. The trial court judge acts as gatekeeper to determine the reliability and credibility of scientific evidence and expert testimony. Also, Federal Rule of Evidence 403 relates to the admissibility of evidence that may cause unfair prejudice. DNA profiling is considered to be a sound technique and is normally admissible in both state and federal courts. The expert witness must be presented as credible and qualified to offer testimony. Also, when producing scientific evidence, the "chain of custody" must be preserved.

LNC's review of evidence

The LNC may be the designated medical investigator in a criminal action, either on behalf of the plaintiff or defendant. In this role, the LNC must have both criminal law and medical knowledge. The LNC may be required to view evidence gathered at the crime scene. This evidence is normally very important, since most of the physical evidence comes from the scene. The evidence from the crime scene will be processed, documented, and placed in custody until needed at any point in the legal procedure. The evidence must be property identified and remain in proper custody if it is to be admitted as evidence at trial. The LNC should also be familiar with forensic science when reviewing a criminal action. These fields include pathology, anthropology, biology, chemistry, serology, toxicology, as well as all additional scientific fields. The LNC may have to work with experts in various scientific fields, so a working knowledge of the field(s) is helpful.

Evidence the LNC may review in criminal actions

The LNC may review medical reports to determine whether the victim's injuries are valid based upon the allegations. The autopsy report will address such items as the extent of

- 130 -

Copyright © Mometrix Media. You have been licensed one copy of this document for personal use only.
Any other reproduction or redistribution is strictly prohibited. All rights reserved.

injuries related to the allegations, pre-existing injuries, gunshot wound information, type of weapon, type of death (e.g., suicide), and the time between the injury and death. Police reports can be reviewed in relation to the medical information, witness identification, and data relative to the responding law enforcement agency. The supplemental investigative reports can also assist relative to witness statements and evidence gathered at the scene or elsewhere. The LNC may review a sexual assault report to determine the injuries sustained and consistency with other report information. Psychological reports may help when determining the validity of plaintiff's allegations or his/her competency. Last, forensic science reports can be utilized to connect a victim and an accused person.

Actions the LNC might investigate
- Child abuse: The LNC should investigate the child's history and current medical information, as well as the family history. The LNC should also determine whether acute injuries have been intentionally inflicted or are accidental. The child's school records should be reviewed, as well as behavioral issues.
- Elder abuse: Elder abuse includes physical and financial abuse, neglect, and self-neglect. The LNC should interview the alleged victim, noting the person's overall health, nutritional state, whether the utilities in the home are operable, and whether the individual has another individual providing case (e.g., housekeeping).
- Domestic violence: Domestic violence emergency response teams (DVERT) are currently being formed in the United States to assist with domestic violence. The LNC should review records to look for previous incidents of violence involving the individual, as well as the medical records of all parties involved. Whether or not children are involved should be determined, and the children's protection should be assured.
- Sexual assault, driving under the influence, and death investigations in which the LNC might be involved for investigation
- Sexual assault: The definition of sexual assault or rape is one party's forced penetration (vulvar, anal, or oral) via penis, object, or body part without the consent of the other party. The LNC investigation should include all 911 information, crime lab reports, evidence, the SART examination, suspect examination report, and health history. Sexual assault can be defended only by alleging the defendant did not commit the act or the victim consented.

Copyright © Mometrix Media. You have been licensed one copy of this document for personal use only. Any other reproduction or redistribution is strictly prohibited. All rights reserved.

- Driving under the influence: This type of investigation is done relative to traffic investigations, driving under the influence citations, diminished capacity defense, and public intoxication issues. Presumption of being under the influence begins at a 0.10% blood alcohol level. The LNC should consider the defendant's physical stature, medical history, and medications (prescription and non-prescription) taken.
- Death investigations: The LNC will not be involved in the investigation conducted by the law enforcement agency, which will include finding the body, determining cause of death, and crime scene review. The LNC, however, must understand different types of death and the manner in which each might occur.

Plea bargaining relative to criminal actions

Plea bargaining involves negotiations to resolve a criminal case without trial. The prosecutor and defendant's attorney negotiate the plea. The plea bargain may occur as late as jury deliberation. The defendant enters a plea to a lesser charge, although the judge retains the right to refuse the plea bargain. Normally, the judge will accept the plea bargain based upon the prosecutor's judgment. Plea bargains negate the expense and time involved in trial. The plea also protects society, since the defendant must accept the consequence of the criminal act to which he/she pleads, although the sentence imposed will likely be less severe than that associated with the original charge.

Copyright © Mometrix Media. You have been licensed one copy of this document for personal use only. Any other reproduction or redistribution is strictly prohibited. All rights reserved.

Administrative

Federal Register

The Federal Register is one of two official federal sources for administrative law. The source is a daily newspaper (Monday through Friday) and contains federal administrative agency information. The agency information includes regulations adopted, regulations being considered, hearing notices regarding proposals, meeting notices and agendas, Executive Orders, and Presidential Proclamations. The agencies are listed in the Register in alphabetical order. The table of contents can be utilized to access the agencies in the newspaper. Also, a monthly index is published which provides up-to-date information regarding regulations and agencies. The Federal Register does not list agencies by responsibility, but only by agency name.

Code of Federal Regulations

The Code of Federal Regulations (C.F.R.) is an official federal source of administrative law. The Code is preferred over the Federal Register. The C.F.R. organizes fifty agency titles, with chapter, subchapter, part, and section subdivisions. The C.F.R. resembles the United States Code, but the titles contained in the sources may not necessarily coincide. The C.F.R. has a life of the agencies and each corresponding title in the back of each volume. To research agencies by topic, however, the researcher must know the agency responsible for the particular topic. An example of a regulation citation might be: 22 C.F.R. pt. 103 (1992), which means the 1992 regulation is found at title 22 of the C.F.R. at part 103, or if not a part but a section, the section symbol would be utilized in the citation instead.

Copyright © Mometrix Media. You have been licensed one copy of this document for personal use only. Any other reproduction or redistribution is strictly prohibited. All rights reserved.

Elder

Geriatric case manager

The geriatric are manager is defined by the National Association of Professional Geriatric Care Managers as an individual "committed to maximizing the independence and autonomy of elders while striving to ensure that the highest quality an most cost-effective health and human services are used where and when appropriate." Depending upon the client, the case manager's responsibilities will fluctuate. At times, the case manager may work with a client living with family members. When a client lives with his/her family, the case manager must be cognizant of the family's role and interaction with the client. At other times, the case manager may work with a client whose family members do not reside in the same area. When the client's family resides in another city or state, the family may depend upon the case manager to advise them of possible issues or situations the care manager feels might occur.

Case manager

In addition to ordinary and general case management responsibilities, the elderly may also need help with eligibility issues, legal matters, and insurance claims or problems. The case manager's ability to evaluate the elderly client's physical abilities, family and friend network, and financial means may allow the client to remain in his/her home, rather than being relocated to a retirement or nursing home. To properly evaluate the client's needs and abilities, it is helpful for the case manager to meet with all members of the client's network. The case manager can then assess the conflicts that can disrupt the elderly client's ability to obtain care or care for him/herself, or to determine those individuals who can assist in client care. The case manager should also be certain the client understands all issues, since it is the goal of the case manager to allow the client to make his/her own decisions. If the case manager feels the client requires asset or physical protection, the case manager should take appropriate steps to insure such care.

Copyright © Mometrix Media. You have been licensed one copy of this document for personal use only. Any other reproduction or redistribution is strictly prohibited. All rights reserved.

Employment Issues

Nurse's Bill of Rights

Pursuant to M. Chenevert's Pro-Nurse Handbook, 2nd Edition, a nurse has the right to:

- be treated with respect;
- expect a reasonable workload;
- an equitable wage;
- the ability to set his/her own priorities;
- ask for what he/she wants;
- refuse a request without an excuse or feeling guilt;
- make errors and take responsibility for mistakes;
- give and receive information as a professional;
- act in a manner perceived as in the best interest of a patient;
- be human.

Facility liability

- Respondeat superior is the first recognized legal responsibility of a facility relative to its employees and their acts. Two other areas of liability include ostensible authority, which involves independent contractors, and corporate negligence, which pertains to hiring qualified individuals and responsibly supervising employees. Respondeat superior involves liability as a result of an act or omission of an employee which occurs during, and within the scope of, employment.
- Ostensible authority involves liability when a patient suffers injury as a result of the negligence of a physician or nurse when the patient expects treatment from the facility as a result of a physician or nurse assigned by the facility.
- Corporate negligence involves liability when a physician or nurse provides substandard care, and the facility knew, or should have known, the outcome of the care.

Copyright © Mometrix Media. You have been licensed one copy of this document for personal use only. Any other reproduction or redistribution is strictly prohibited. All rights reserved.

Ostensible authority or agency doctrine

If the patient reasonably believes an independent contractor is an employee of a facility, the facility may be liable for the contractor's negligence. In order to establish ostensible authority, the courts require the presence of the following elements: subjective, inherent function, reliance, and control. The subjective test involves whether the patient looked to the facility for treatment and was treated by a health care provider acting as an ostensible agent. The inherent function test normally applies to emergency treatment, when the independent contractor physician provides care as an inherent function of the facility. With reliance, the facility may be held liable if a patient suffers injuries as a result of a facility's acts or omissions while the patient is relying upon the judgment of the facility. Control by the facility may be determined if the facility maintains some control over the independent contractor, including such elements as the type of occupation, if facility personnel normally supervise the contractor, who supplies the workplace and instruments, and payment method.

Corporate negligence and negligent hiring

With corporate negligence, a facility may be found liable for failure to hire qualified employees and/or failure to properly supervise employee performance. With negligent hiring, the facility may be found liable for failure to check references, a criminal record, license status, skills, and education. A physician's and an advance practice nurse's credentials should also be confirmed. The facility may check credentials through the National Practitioner Data Bank and the Health Care Integrity and Protection Data Bank. The facility is also responsible for supervising personnel, whether employees or independent contractors. The facility is also responsible for maintaining the appropriate standard of care. The facility may suffer liability if an employee is not terminated under the "failure to fire" policy.

NPDB and HIP DB

The National Practitioner Data Bank (NPDB) was established in 1990. The NPDB acts as a central storehouse for state actions relative to licensed health care practitioners. The NPDB is designed to take care of issues that may arise as a result of health care providers who move out of a state to practice in another state, when the practitioner has lost his/her

Copyright © Mometrix Media. You have been licensed one copy of this document for personal use only. Any other reproduction or redistribution is strictly prohibited. All rights reserved.

license or facility privileges or is subject to discipline by a facility or state license board. All actions taken by a state or licensing board must be reported to the NPDB, and the information is available to any facility that requests information. The Health Care Integrity and Protection Data Bank (HIP-DB) represent flagging systems designed to allow complete reviews relative to health care providers. The purpose of the HIP-DB is to negate fraud and abuse in the health care system. The HIP-DB maintains records relative to health care related criminal convictions, judgments, federal and state health care program exclusion proceedings, and license and certification actions.

Employment at will vs. contract employment

Normally, employment is "at will," wherein no written contract specifies the terms of employment. In the case of "at will" employment, the employee or the employer may terminate employment without cause or notice. Some higher level nurses may be employed under a written contract. If a contract exists, the employee cannot be terminated or discharged before expiration of the contract or the employer may be subject to liability. The contract normally sets forth terms of termination. If the contract does not specify terms, the employee may be terminated only if the contract has expired or the employee breaches the terms of the contract.

Contract entered into after employment

Employment contracts after employment commences may include handbooks or personnel/policy manuals. Language in the handbook or manual can supersede employment at will. Three theories normally apply to ascertain whether the handbook or manual is considered a contract. First, the employees' expectations are considered. Second, the employees' and employer's expectations may be considered. Third, a unilateral contract may be determined to exist. Handbooks or manuals may be amended by employers, and the amendment should be designated as a "restatement." A written statement should be signed by the employee to confirm receipt of the notice. Vague words, such as satisfactory or reasonable, may be interpreted differently by an employee and the courts.

Copyright © Mometrix Media. You have been licensed one copy of this document for personal use only. Any other reproduction or redistribution is strictly prohibited. All rights reserved.

Independent consideration relative to employment

Many courts will not uphold an employment contract if the policies of an employer include disclaimers asserting the procedures do not embody an employment contract. Rather, the disclaimer is normally upheld by the court. The employer can state that the contents of the employee manual or handbook do not represent an employment relationship or contract. The manual or handbook may also be changed by the employer when he/she/it reserves the right to do so. On the other hand, an employee who receives extra or independent consideration over and above that stated in an employment contract, such as a bonus or additional benefits, the employer may not be entitled to terminate the employee at will. This provision may apply even if the contract or policies seem to designate an at will relationship.

Two exceptions to at will employment

The major exceptions to at will employment include "public policy" and "implied covenant of good faith and fair dealing." With public policy, the employee is protected from at will termination when the reason for termination does not coincide with accepted public policy. This exception includes termination as a result of assertion of a statutory right, following the law, or refusing to perform an act prohibited by law. This exception also includes the "whistle-blower" laws. Under implied covenant of good faith and fair dealing, the employee cannot be terminated in an effort to deprive him/her of earned compensation. Many courts recognize employment relations as an obligation between employer and employee, negating the employer's ability to terminate the employee simply to deprive him/her of compensation that has already been earned but not received, such as a commission.

Definitions

- Defamation: The public ridicule or contempt suffered by a party as a result of oral or written publication of untrue statements by another party constitutes defamation.
- Conditional privilege: When a previous employer discloses derogatory statements (possibly regarding the employee's character and abilities) to a former employee's prospective employer, the former employer may not be liable for the statements pursuant to conditional privilege.

Copyright © Mometrix Media. You have been licensed one copy of this document for personal use only. Any other reproduction or redistribution is strictly prohibited. All rights reserved.

- Loss of conditional privilege: When an employer negligently distributes statements, untruths, non-verified information, or error-free data regarding an employee, the employee can claim loss of conditional privilege, subjecting the employer to liability.
- Sexual harassment: Sexual harassment involves two types: quid pro quo and hostile environment. Sexual harassment deals with the abuse of power and control over employees in "lower" positions, specifically if submission is a condition of continued employment, interferes with the employee's work performance, becomes a basis for decisions regarding the employee, or a hostile or threatening environment results.

ADA

In 1990, the Americans with Disabilities Act (ADA) was passed. The Act is designed to negate all employment discrimination against Americans with either mental or physical disabilities. The Act is also designed to allow equal opportunities, participation in activities, and economic self-support for disabled Americans. The Americans with Disabilities Act defines "disability" as "any physical or mental impairment that limits any major life activity." The Act includes obvious disabilities, as well as abilities not apparent, such as diabetes or AIDS. The Act also covers a person who has a relationship with a disabled party. Illegal drug use is not covered by the Act. Homosexuals, bisexuals, transvestites, transsexuals, pedophiles, exhibitionists, voyeurs, gender identity disorders, gamblers, pyromaniacs, and kleptomaniacs are omitted from coverage.

<u>Work environment and prospective employers</u>
As a result of the Americans with Disabilities Act, most employers no longer require medical inquiries prior to employment, and questionnaires regarding medical information have been altered to discard information about previous injuries, employment compensation claims, and diseases. Employers cannot question a prospective employee about the nature of his/her disability. A medical examination required as a basis for employment must be related to the job in question. The employer must state the functions of a prospective job and must then determine whether the prospective employee is qualified for the position (with or without reasonable accommodation) and confirm that the prospective employee would not pose a threat to others in the workplace. The

Copyright © Mometrix Media. You have been licensed one copy of this document for personal use only. Any other reproduction or redistribution is strictly prohibited. All rights reserved.

employee is considered qualified if he/she is able to safely perform the functions of the job. Employers must educate employees regarding the Act's requirements.

Defenses to Americans with Disabilities Act claims

- Undue hardship clause: If a reasonable accommodation for a disabled employee is expensive or difficult to accomplish, an employer may claim undue hardship. The employer must explore options prior to making the determination that accommodation is expensive or difficult.
- Qualification standard and health and safety defense: The inability of an employee to safely perform job-related tasks or when the safety of other employees may be affected, an employer may claim this defense.
- Religious entities defense: Prospective employers who are religious entities may give preference to prospective employees of a specific religion.
- Public safety defense: The inability of an employer to provide reasonable accommodation that will protect others from infectious or communicable diseases can offer a public safety defense.

Copyright © Mometrix Media. You have been licensed one copy of this document for personal use only. Any other reproduction or redistribution is strictly prohibited. All rights reserved.

Contracts

Definitions

- Merger clause: This clause in a contract reflects the final agreement between the parties to the contract, indicating changes to the contract require a written document signed and dated by all original parties, specifically stating the modification is to become a part of the original contract.

- Duty to mitigate: When included in a contract, this clause requires an injured party to attempt to decrease the damages. For instance, in a wrongful discharge action, the injured party may be required to actively pursue other employment and the damages may be reduced by the earnings of the injured party.

- Restitution: If an injured party receives comparable property or a monetary award equal to the loss, this is an act of restitution by the defendant.

- Facilitation: Facilitation involves gathering parties to a dispute together for a meeting before a facilitator with the intention of resolving issues between the parties.

- Facilitator: If facilitation occurs, the facilitator is the neutral party overseeing the discussions between parties to a dispute. The facilitator's role is to develop organization and discussion in an effort to resolve all or part of a dispute.

- Summary jury trial: The summary jury trial is designed to offer the parties involved in a dispute an opportunity to view strengths and weaknesses of each party's action. The proceeding is a condensed trial held in a private setting.

Role of the independent contractor

An independent contractor's role is to perform a particular job for another individual, company, or facility. In performing the job, the independent contractor utilizes his/her individual means and methods, with no authority exercised by the individual, company, or facility retaining him/her. The main indication that an individual is an independent contractor is the scope of control. The independent contractor normally lacks the ability to provide training or instruct others, he/she may provide work for others as well, and he/she may utilize personal tools and hire any individuals necessary to perform the job for which hired. Also, independent contractors do not normally maintain specific hours and may not

Copyright © Mometrix Media. You have been licensed one copy of this document for personal use only.
Any other reproduction or redistribution is strictly prohibited. All rights reserved.

be required to work at the retaining employer's site. The contractor cannot terminate employment, and the retaining employer cannot fire him/her. The contractor may complete the project in an order tailored to his/her liking. Compensation is based upon the specific job, agreed commission, or a specific period (hourly, weekly, etc.). The independent contractor is responsible for his/her own expenses, although he/she can bill for expenses if agreed upon between the parties.

Elements of an independent contractor contract

To be considered a binding, valid contract, the independent contractor contract must contain certain elements. The document should specifically identify all parties to the contract, setting out full names, addresses, and titles. The body of the contract should state the owner's business type and a comprehensive set of terms and conditions under which the contractor is being retained. The type of work to be performed should be described. The compensation to be paid should be specifically noted, including all schedules of payment. The independent contractor's liability insurance information should be included. The contract period should be specifically set forth, including a start date and end date. The independent status of the contractor should be noted in the contract, specifically indicating the contractor is not an employee of the retaining party. The contract may also contain alternative dispute resolution language. Last, the document should be signed and dated by each party entering into the agreement.

Role and elements of the consultant

The consultant is normally retained to provide advice to the retaining party. In some instances, the consultant may also perform work at the employer's site or another location. The consulting contract should contain certain elements to protect the parties. The full name, address, and titles for each party should be clearly stated in the contract. The consultant's responsibilities should also be clearly stated, concentrating on the consulting duties. The consultant's workplace site should be included, whether at the employer's workplace or an independent location. The period of time for performance under the contract should be stated, including the compensation to be paid/received. The compensation should include reimbursement for out-of-pocket costs. The contract may contain a non-compete clause restricting the work a consultant may enter into during the term of the contract; this is negotiable. The contract may also contain alternative dispute resolution language.

Copyright © Mometrix Media. You have been licensed one copy of this document for personal use only. Any other reproduction or redistribution is strictly prohibited. All rights reserved.

Nursing Practice

Nursing licensure

The process through which a nurse obtains permission to engage in the nursing practice is licensure through an agency of a state government. The nurse must demonstrate that he/she has a required level of competency. The start of regulation of nurse licensure began after the early 1990s. Thereafter, use of the title "nurse" and the practice of nursing were regulated by laws. The laws regulated requirements for practice and penalties. Licensing is granted in two forms: mandatory or permissive. With mandatory licensing, the nurse must comply with licensing statutes if he/she practices within the sphere of the nursing profession. With permissive licensing, the nurse must comply with licensing statutes if he/she intends to use the actual title given by the licensing agency (thus, regulating use of the title).

Credentialing

Credentialing is a form of certification. Credentialing involves a voluntary process of self-regulation found in the health care environment. Credentialing indicates that a nurse has complied with higher standards, as opposed to licensure which indicates a nurse has performed minimum competency standards set by a licensing agency. In the health care environment, credentialing provides a means to advance the health care profession, as well as protecting patients. In the health care environment, the standards set normally pertain to subspecialties. Certification is sometimes sought by educational programs and institutions as well. When the program or institution holds certifications, the implication exists that the program or institution has gone beyond the standards of a particular licensing agency.

ANA's Certification Program

The ANA Certification Program was established in 1973. This Program is designed to acknowledge professional achievement relative to specific areas of nursing. The Program was changed to the American Nurses Credentialing Center in 1991. This Center became a

Copyright © Mometrix Media. You have been licensed one copy of this document for personal use only. Any other reproduction or redistribution is strictly prohibited. All rights reserved.

separate corporation whose function is to certify RN and advanced practice nurses in specialty functions. The Open Door 2000 program established by the American Nurses Credentialing Center provides for the two levels of credentialing. These two levels consist of Certified (being RN, C) and Board Certified (being RN, BC). The Open Door 2000 program also provides for criteria for certification, which includes educational preparation, recognized knowledge, skills, and competence as a result of experience.

Definitions

- Certification: This encompasses the RN, C credential. The Committee on Certification for Diploma and Associate Degree Nursing Practice and the Committee on Modular Certificate designate recipients of certification.
- Board-level certification: This encompasses the RN, BC credential. The Board on Certification for Baccalaureate Nursing Practice and the Board on Certification for Advanced Nursing Practice designate recipients of certification.
- Advance practice certification: This encompasses the APRN, BC credential. Advanced practice nurses receive this new credential; the BC can be included to a nurse's designation when required by the nurse's practice state.
- Nursing administration certification: This encompasses the CNA, BC and CNAA, BC credentials.

Prescriptive authority

In the nursing practice, the nurse entitled to prescriptive authority is entitled to prescribe or dispense certain medications or devices, but with limited authority and pursuant to specific protocols. When determining the ability of a nurse to prescribe, the issues of whether the state recognizes the authority and whether the state provides procedures for this authority arise. Several states have, to a limited extent, recognized nurses' prescriptive authority since 1991, normally acknowledging rules established between a nurse and a physician. Many states will allow advanced practice nurses this authority to some extent. Also, the ANA has recommended legislation suggesting caution relative to the authority of a nurse to dispense medication, indicating that the authority should extend only to the doses required by the patient until such time as the prescription can be obtained from a pharmacist.

Copyright © Mometrix Media. You have been licensed one copy of this document for personal use only. Any other reproduction or redistribution is strictly prohibited. All rights reserved.

Disciplinary actions

Disciplinary action is established pursuant to the traditional disciplinary system. Pursuant to this system, the state board is entitled to take action relative to a nursing license when alleged violations occur, including reinstatement of licenses. The disciplinary actions the nurse may be subject to include a license being denied, revoked, or suspended; a probationary period being set; or conditions placed upon the license (e.g., psychiatric evaluation). In the event of a disciplinary action, the nurse is entitled to certain rights before, during, and after the proceeding. The nurse is entitled to notice of the time and place of the hearing, representation by an attorney, and a concise statement of the charges against the nurse. The nurse is also entitled to confrontation of witnesses, production of witnesses on his/her behalf, and the record or transcript of the proceeding. The determination by the individual or panel of individuals must be fair based upon the evidence presented, and the nurse has the right to appeal the decision or request judicial review.

Copyright © Mometrix Media. You have been licensed one copy of this document for personal use only. Any other reproduction or redistribution is strictly prohibited. All rights reserved.

Practice Test

Practice Questions

1. When screening a medical-related case, which of the following cases is most likely to result in low damages, for which a plaintiff attorney may reject a case?
   a. Vision impairment related to chronic use of corticosteroids
   b. Birth injury resulting in cerebral palsy
   c. Incorrect diagnosis of cancer, resulting in delayed treatment
   d. Medication error resulting in renal failure

2. A customer slips and falls on a wet floor in a department store, resulting in a vertebral fracture and sues for damages. This type of case is classified as
   a. environmental case.
   b. medical malpractice
   c. general negligence.
   d. workplace injury.

3. As part of a marketing strategy to attract new clients, the CLNC plans to offer a discount for first-time clients. Which of the following is a reasonable discount?
   a. First case at no charge
   b. Ten percent discount for first case
   c. Fifty percent discount for first case
   d. Individually negotiated discount

4. Which of the following is an example of a strict liability crime, which does not require a *mens reus*?
   a. Statutory rape
   b. Sexual assault
   c. Medicare fraud
   d. Possession of narcotics with intent to sell

5. A written report should be completed for
   a. all cases evaluated by the CLNC.
   b. only those cases deemed meritorious or defensible.
   c. only those cases for which the client attorney requests a written report.
   d. only those cases in which the CLNC serves as a testifying expert.

Copyright © Mometrix Media. You have been licensed one copy of this document for personal use only. Any other reproduction or redistribution is strictly prohibited. All rights reserved.

6. Which of the following is true regarding a CLNC serving as a testifying expert?
    a. The CLNC is expected to prepare attorneys and help with the case.
    b. The CLNC may review all aspects of a case, even those outside of professional expertise.
    c. Work products, such as notes, are not discoverable.
    d. Work products, such as notes, may be discoverable.

7. A worker falls from a ladder during employment, resulting in a fractured femur; however, the worker failed to follow standard safety procedures. The worker is receiving benefits under Worker's Compensation but wishes to file suit against the employer for pain and suffering. Which of the following is correct?
    a. The employer is immune from further liability.
    b. The employer is liable and may be sued.
    c. The worker may lose all Workers' Compensation benefits upon bringing suit.
    d. The worker should not have received Worker's Compensation benefits.

8. Which type of evidence is derived from a patient's medical records?
    a. Testimonial
    b. Physical/real
    c. Hearsay
    d. Demonstrative

9. Which of the following legal procedures authorizes disclosure of patient personal health information?
    a. Subpoena
    b. Subpoena duces tecum
    c. Warrant
    d. Court order

10. Which of the following is the best response during a court proceeding when the attorney for the defense asks if the CLNC is a "victim advocate?"
    a. "Yes."
    b. "No."
    c. "I advocate for all patients."
    d. "I'm not sure what you mean."

11. Which of the following is within the scope of practice of a CLNC?
    a. Providing legal advice
    b. Advocating a position
    c. Speaking for a patient
    d. Providing nursing opinions

Copyright © Mometrix Media. You have been licensed one copy of this document for personal use only. Any other reproduction or redistribution is strictly prohibited. All rights reserved.

12. When providing a promotional packet to a potential client, which of the following should the CLNC include in the packet?
   a. Sample of work product
   b. Schedule of fees
   c. List of previous clients
   d. Summary of previous cases

13. When researching, for which of the following would the CLNC find Worker' Compensation data most useful?
   a. Tracking occupational illness
   b. Determining safety measures
   c. Estimating frequency of particular occupational injuries
   d. Reducing costs of work-related injuries

14. Which of the following is correct regarding civil actions?
   a. Action is considered a crime against society as a whole.
   b. Verdict requires unanimous agreement by jury.
   c. Penalty does not involve monetary damages.
   d. Proof must be by preponderance of the evidence.

15. The CLNC is hired by a plaintiff's attorney to interview the plaintiff regarding his upcoming testimony. During the interview, the CLNC finds that the plaintiff is making exaggerated and untruthful claims about the injury. The CLNC's duty is to
   a. confront the plaintiff.
   b. notify the plaintiff's attorney of the findings.
   c. notify the defendant's attorney.
   d. notify the insurance company.

16. The CLNC conducts the pre-litigation phase of a potential lawsuit by interviewing the potential defendant and reviewing the incident report. Which of the following is of most concern?
   a. The potential defendant filled out the incident report two weeks after the event, when the plaintiff complained of persistent pain.
   b. The incident report included an addendum with notes about conversations with the potential plaintiff after the event.
   c. The incident report contained the names of witnesses and their statements, but not their signatures.
   d. The incident report was misfiled and unavailable for review until found 2 days later.

17. The first step in evaluating whether a health care practitioner has complied with standards of care is to
   a. do a survey of the scientific literature regarding standards of care.
   b. access the appropriate state practice act, such as the Board of Nursing Practice Act.
   c. gather information from professional associations.
   d. review organization/agency/facility policies and procedures.

Copyright © Mometrix Media. You have been licensed one copy of this document for personal use only. Any other reproduction or redistribution is strictly prohibited. All rights reserved.

18. What is the name for the phase of litigation during which the complaint is filed?
    a. Pleading
    b. Trial/arbitration
    c. Discovery
    d. Pre-litigation

19. When determining the burden of proof for acts of negligence, how would the CLNC classify willfully providing inadequate care while disregarding safety and security?
    a. Negligent conduct
    b. Gross negligence
    c. Contributory negligence
    d. Comparative negligence

20. When screening for medical-related cases, what are the four necessary elements of negligence claims?
    a. Duty to care, harm, liability, and residual
    b. Onset, duration, cause, and injury
    c. Victim, perpetrator, injury, and residual
    d. Duty of care, breach of duty, damages, and causation

21. When locating a testifying expert for the plaintiff, which information should be shared initially to rule out a conflict of interest?
    a. A detailed outline of the case, including the merits of the plaintiff's case
    b. A summary of documents and records
    c. Names of parties involved, significant players and facilities, and insurance companies
    d. Names of parties involved (plaintiffs and defendants) only

22. A consulting expert's notes and opinions regarding a case are discoverable when the
    a. consulting expert is one of only a dozen experts on the subject.
    b. consulting expert's opinions and notes were used by the testifying expert to form an opinion.
    c. consulting expert has provided a written document detailing weaknesses of the case.
    d. opposing attorney consults expert's notes and opinions.

23. Which of the following is an example of a products liability case?
    a. Severe adverse reaction to a drug
    b. Exposure to hazardous chemicals in the work environment
    c. Physician delay of treatment
    d. Failure of insurance company to pay claims

Copyright © Mometrix Media. You have been licensed one copy of this document for personal use only. Any other reproduction or redistribution is strictly prohibited. All rights reserved.

24. Which of the following is the method of discovery that involves sending a list of questions from one party to a second party, requesting that the second party respond under oath in writing?
    a. Deposition
    b. Request for production of documents
    c. Interrogatory
    d. Request for admission

25. What is an example of an intentional tort?
    a. A nurse fails to observe adverse effects after administering a medication.
    b. A shed containing toxic chemicals explodes, exposing nearby residents.
    c. A physician administers a blood product to a Jehovah's Witness despite explicit refusal by patient.
    d. A person swinging a bat during a baseball game loses grip, and the bat injures a bystander.

26. When initially screening a medical-related plaintiff case to determine if it is meritorious, what should the CLNC focus on?
    a. Strengths of the case
    b. Weaknesses of the case
    c. Extent of injury
    d. Availability of testifying expert

27. Following discovery but pre-trial, the parties in a dispute agree to sit down with a third party (a judge) to try to reach a voluntary settlement. What is this type of alternative dispute resolution (ADR) called?
    a. Arbitration
    b. Mini-trial
    c. Summary trial
    d. Mediation

28. A client experiences a severe reaction to the formaldehyde fumes in a carpet installed in the home and is suing the manufacturer for medical damages. This type of case is classified as
    a. criminal.
    b. general negligence.
    c. toxic tort.
    d. product liability.

29. When screening medical records for tampering, which of the following should be an alert?
    a. There is a mismatch in the ink color from one part of an entry to another.
    b. The medical report does not include billing statements.
    c. The MRI report does not include films.
    d. The incident report is missing from the medical record.

Copyright © Mometrix Media. You have been licensed one copy of this document for personal use only. Any other reproduction or redistribution is strictly prohibited. All rights reserved.

30. When preparing a written report of a medical malpractice case that involves extensive medical terminology, what is the best practice?
 a. Include a vocabulary list with definitions in an addendum.
 b. Ask the client/attorney if he or she needs definitions.
 c. Place definitions in footnotes.
 d. Place definitions in parentheses following terms in the body of the report.

31. Which theory of vicarious liability applies when an employer is considered directly responsible for negligence of its employees toward clients?
 a. Employer's liability
 b. *Respondeat superior*
 c. Ostensible agency
 d. Direct corporate liability

32. Which of the following cases would most likely be rejected by a plaintiff attorney?
 a. An 80-year-old patient suffered postoperative complications but recovered fully.
 b. Brain damage occurred following complications after colon resection.
 c. Malignant tumor was misdiagnosed and a 50-year old patient died.
 d. An infant died after premature birth in which no neonatologist was in attendance.

33. Which of the following is the most important assurance that a forensic document examiner (FDE) will be an effective testifying expert to identify authors of documents to be entered as evidence?
 a. The FDE advertises services as a "graphologist."
 b. The FDE has testified in previous trials.
 c. The FDE is certified by the American Board of Forensic Document Examiners (ABFDE).
 d. The FDE is a member of the American Association of Handwriting Analysts (AAHA).

34. In a state in which the tort of intentional spoliation is not recognized but the defendant destroyed evidence, what is the primary purpose of presenting evidence that the destruction occurred?
 a. To prevent the defendant from destroying more evidence
 b. To provide impetus for a change in the law to recognize intentional spoliation
 c. To establish a basis for further legal action
 d. To strengthen the case for the plaintiff

35. Which of the following is the best research approach to finding an expert witness for a specific disorder?
 a. Use survey textbooks.
 b. Use the Internet to access online journals.
 c. Use Internet databases to find authors with multiple articles or entries.
 d. Search reference collections.

Copyright © Mometrix Media. You have been licensed one copy of this document for personal use only. Any other reproduction or redistribution is strictly prohibited. All rights reserved.

36. If an attorney for a plaintiff is arguing that an adverse effect occurred following an innovative treatment because standards of care (SOC) were not followed, the best argument for the defense might be that standards of care
    a. don't yet reflect current cutting-edge medical treatments.
    b. don't apply to this case.
    c. are too general to be used to quantify treatment.
    d. were followed to the extent possible.

37. When assessing whether a managed care organization (MCO) is guilty of negligent utilization review, which of the following types of utilization review has the highest potential for liability?
    a. Concurrent
    b. Prospective
    c. Retrospective
    d. Terminal

38. The National Committee for Quality Assurance (NCQA) has how many levels of accreditation for managed care organizations (MCOs)?
    a. 6
    b. 4
    c. 3
    d. 5

39. What type of request directed to plaintiffs for production includes the product alleged to have caused injury?
    a. Medical
    b. Witnesses
    c. General
    d. Financial

40. A financial request for production directed to defendants would likely include
    a. medical bills.
    b. tax returns:
    c. withholding forms.
    d. insurance policies.

41. When preparing demonstrative evidence to support a plaintiff's claim resulting from injuries incurred in an auto accident in which the defendant struck the plaintiff's car after the defendant ran a red light and made an illegal left-hand turn, what is the best medium to use?
    a. Photo of the accident
    b. Recording of the 911 call
    c. Computer-generated animation
    d. Hand-drawn illustration on a flipchart

Copyright © Mometrix Media. You have been licensed one copy of this document for personal use only.
Any other reproduction or redistribution is strictly prohibited. All rights reserved.

42. The CLNC has reviewed medical records as a consulting expert and must interface with a testifying expert (TE) in order to provide the TE materials. What is the most appropriate method to ensure that the TE reviews the material that supports the client?
    a. Underline or highlight select information in documents provided.
    b. Provide an addendum that lists the documents and line numbers of select information.
    c. Provide a summary that describes the supporting material.
    d. Deliver the materials to the TE for review.

43. When the CLNC is serving as a testifying witness for the plaintiff, the opposing attorney attacks the CLNC's credibility by asking if the CLNC is being paid to testify, suggesting the CLNC is a "hired gun." Which of the following is the best response?
    a. "I'm not biased against the defendant."
    b. "I don't take every case, just those I believe have merit."
    c. "All expert witnesses are reimbursed for their time."
    d. "My pay has nothing to do with the merits of the case."

44. When assessing the qualifications of a testifying expert for a case that involved a general practitioner's misdiagnosis of a patient with a brain tumor, which of the following testifying experts would likely be the best choice?
    a. A practicing board-certified neurosurgeon
    b. A nurse with experience in neurology
    c. A retired general practitioner
    d. A non-practicing, board-certified neurosurgeon who serves only as an expert witness

45. In which clause of a contract would the fee for the consulting services that the CLNC is to receive be outlined?
    a. Expenses
    b. Notices
    c. Definitions
    d. Consideration

46. Prior to signing a contract with a client, what is the CLNC's most important step?
    a. Personally review the entire contract.
    b. Hire an attorney specializing in contracts to review the contract.
    c. Clarify inconsistencies in a letter agreement.
    d. Review the entire contract with the client.

47. A CLNC is accused of malpractice and under the element of causation, the attorney for the plaintiff attempts to prove that the actions of the CLNC were the primary cause of damages. This test of negligence is referred to as
    a. but for.
    b. foreseeability.
    c. substantial factor.
    d. *res ipsa loquitur.*

Copyright © Mometrix Media. You have been licensed one copy of this document for personal use only. Any other reproduction or redistribution is strictly prohibited. All rights reserved.

48. Which of the following actions could result in a CLNC being accused of practicing law without a license?

    a. The CLNC prepares a list of client questions about the case and gives it to the attorney for response.

    b. The CLNC advises the client that the statute of limitations on an action will expire in 6 months.

    c. The in-house CLNC communicates legal advice from the attorney to the client.

    d. The in-house CLNC signs letters on behalf of the attorney as a legal nurse consultant.

49. Which of the following is a good interview strategy?

    a. Write a script and thoroughly learn the content.

    b. Write and memorize, word-for-word, a script.

    c. Outline a script and refer to the outline during the interview.

    d. Present a PowerPoint presentation of the scripted material during the interview.

50. When requesting a plaintiff's medical records from a hospital, the purpose of requesting a certified copy is to ensure that

    a. the administrator of records has certified the patient's medical records as complete.

    b. all patient records and products have been placed in the medical records.

    c. no further discovery related to medical records is necessary.

    d. no alterations have been made in the medical records.

Copyright © Mometrix Media. You have been licensed one copy of this document for personal use only. Any other reproduction or redistribution is strictly prohibited. All rights reserved.

Answers and Explanations

1. A: Vision impairment related to chronic use of corticosteroids is a low damages case and hard to prove negligence. This is because the impact on vision is well known and must be balanced against the need for corticosteroids to treat symptoms related to disease. High damages cases include those in which the direct damage is more evident, such as birth injuries, incorrect diagnosis, and errors in prescription and/or administration of medications. Even if a low damages case has merit, an attorney may feel the return is not worth the time that must be invested.

2. C: General negligence involves nonprofessional personal injury, such as may occur with premises liability, injuries resulting from falls, assaults, excessive drinking, and accidents. Environmental case includes injuries that result from environmental toxins, such as secondary smoke, radiation, asbestos, and toxic chemicals. Medical malpractice involves negligence on the part of a health care provider or those who control access to care. Workplace injury includes injuries that result from employment, such as back injuries and equipment-related injuries.

3. B: A 10%discount is reasonable. Offering to provide free services or a large discount devalues the professional contribution of the CLNC and is often not financially feasible. Professionals usually do not negotiate fees but rely on a fee schedule. Fees should not be contingent on the outcome of the case but should be based on the hours needed to complete a case. The CLNC should always remain professional but firm about fees, stressing the value derived from the CLNC's service.

4. A: Statutory rape does not require a *mens reus* ("guilty mind" or intent to commit a crime) to be considered a criminal act. Even if the person charged believed that the minor involved was of age, this is not considered an excuse to commit the illegal act. In this type of case, the prosecution is not required to prove intent because the crime is self-evident based on its nature. Strict liability cases can include vagrancy, traffic violations, and driving under the influence of drugs or alcohol.

5. C: A written report, including the case report or summary, should only be completed at the request of the attorney. Testifying experts should not complete a written report because this report may be discoverable. When requested, the type of report should be agreed upon between the CNLC and the client attorney. Reports may vary in structure and length with brief reports usually 1 to 15 pages, moderate reports 16 to 50 pages, and comprehensive reports over 50 pages.

6. D: A testifying expert is subject to discovery, so any work products, such as notes, may be discoverable. Generally, a consulting expert is not subject to discovery. A testifying expert must testify only within the person's professional expertise, but a consulting expert may

Copyright © Mometrix Media. You have been licensed one copy of this document for personal use only. Any other reproduction or redistribution is strictly prohibited. All rights reserved.

consult about any aspect of the case, even those outside the person's professional expertise. Experts testify in court while consultants do not, so consultants may help prepare attorneys for the court proceedings.

7. A: In Worker's Compensation, the employer is, with few exceptions, immune from further liability because accepting benefits generally incudes waiving the right to sue. Worker's Compensation regulations may vary somewhat from one state to another. In some states, if the injury resulted from intentional or reckless action on the part of the employer, then the employer may be liable, but in this case, the worker failed to follow standard safety procedures and was, therefore, complicit in the injury.

8. C: Medical records are generally considered hearsay evidence because they often contain entries from multiple departments (admissions, ED, laboratory, unit) and individuals (physicians, nurses, technicians), and bringing all of the contributors to court is not feasible. However, the records may be admissible under the business record exemption or the official document exemption with a custodian as witness to explain the procedures for recordkeeping. It is especially important that all standard procedures for documenting and maintaining medical records are followed.

9. D: A court order authorizes disclosure of a patient's personal health information. In some cases, this court order may cover only restricted information rather than an entire health record. A subpoena is issued to advise a person that he or she must give testimony in court or in a deposition. A subpoena *duces tecum* is similar but requires the person bring specific documents to court. A warrant authorizes an action, such as a search.

10. B: This is a yes/no question, so the correct response is "No." While, in fact, a CLNC may present evidence in support of a plaintiff's case, a victim advocate has a specific role separate from that of the CLNC. A victim advocate may help the person navigate the legal system as well as make referrals to community agencies and service that may benefit the person. The victim advocate often accompanies a person to legal proceedings to provide emotional support.

11. D: The CLNC may provide nursing opinions about health, health care, and injury-related matters but does not speak directly for a patient or advocate for a position. The CLNC must remain objective and provide information, speaking for the profession. The CLNC may not provide any legal advice because this is within the scope of practice of the attorney. The CLNCs scope of practice may vary depending upon whether the person is serving as a testifying or consulting expert; the consulting expert has fewer limitations.

12. A: The promotional packet should include a high-quality brochure that looks professional and outlines services. The packet should not include lists of previous clients or summaries of previous cases since these may involve breach of confidentiality. The schedule of fees should not be included in the packet initially but should be discussed at a later time. Other important elements of the promotional packet include a printed envelope, business cards, introduction letter, and letters of recommendation.

Copyright © Mometrix Media. You have been licensed one copy of this document for personal use only. Any other reproduction or redistribution is strictly prohibited. All rights reserved.

13. C: Workers' Compensation data are not available on a national basis and criteria for data collection may vary from state to state along with state regulations, but even limited (statewide) data may provide an estimate of the frequency and severity of particular occupational injuries as well as associated costs. The data may help guide institution of work safety measures and development of safety training. Occupational illness data are less useful because injuries tend to be similar across industries while illnesses show more variation.

14. D: Proof in civil cases is by preponderance of the evidence rather the criminal case standard of beyond a reasonable doubt. Civil verdicts require a majority agreement by the jury while criminal cases require unanimous agreement. Civil cases, such as those involving personal injury, may include monetary damages while criminal cases generally involve punishment, such as incarceration and/or restitution. Civil actions are considered personal while criminal actions, such as those involving specific crimes like homicide, are considered crimes against society as whole.

15. B: In this case, the CLNC must report the findings to the plaintiff's attorney because the CLNC was hired by the attorney. The CLNC should neither confront the plaintiff nor show disbelief but should appear neutral and gain as much information as possible. The CLNC should try, through questioning, to identify the plaintiff's motives in filing an action against the defendant. Notifying the insurance company or the defendant's attorney would be a violation of privileged communication since the nurse is serving as the attorney's representative.

16. A: The incident report should have been completed immediately after the event. Waiting to write the incident report until the potential plaintiff complains of injury suggests that the incident report may not accurately reflect the events as they occurred. The potential defendant should note in the records any communications with the possible plaintiff about the event. As long as the names and statements of witnesses are contained in the incident report and they can verify that their statements are correct, signatures are usually not required of all witnesses. Misfiling should not affect the case.

17. B: The first step in evaluating standards of care should be to access the appropriate state practice act, such as the Pharmacy Practice Act, Nursing Practice Act, or Medical Practice Act, as these sources outline the scope of practice and standards of care. Practice acts vary somewhat from state to state, so the scopes of practice may differ from one state to another. State and federal laws also provide information about standards of care. Additional information may be gained from regulatory agencies, professional associations, facility sources, literature search, and expert testimony.

18. A: The complaint is filed during the pleading phase. Phases include:
Pre-litigation: Incident reviewed, attorney chosen, power of attorney and contracts signed.
Pleading: Complaint filed by plaintiff and answer, motion, or demurrer filed by defendant.
Discovery: Evidence exchanged.

Copyright © Mometrix Media. You have been licensed one copy of this document for personal use only. Any other reproduction or redistribution is strictly prohibited. All rights reserved.

Trial/Arbitration: Evidence found during discovery regarding complaint presented and refuted with the burden of proof on the plaintiff.

Post-litigation: Attempts made to enforce judgment. This may include hiring others to make collection, garnishing wages, and levying bank accounts. Appeals may be filed.

19. B: Gross negligence. Negligence indicates that *proper care* has not been provided, based on established standards. *Reasonable care* uses rationale for decision-making in relation to providing care. Negligent conduct indicates that an individual failed to provide reasonable care or to protect/assist another, based on standards and expertise. Gross negligence is willfully providing inadequate care while disregarding the safety and security of another. Contributory negligence involves the injured party contributing to his/her own harm. Comparative negligence attempts to determine what percentage amount of negligence is attributed to each individual involved.

20. D: When screening for medical-related cases for plaintiffs, the four necessary elements of negligence must be identified:

Duty of care: The defendant had a duty to provide adequate care and/or protect the plaintiff's safety.

Breach of duty: The defendant failed to carry out the duty to care, resulting in danger, injury, or harm to the plaintiff.

Damages: The plaintiff experienced illness or injury as a result of the breach of duty.

Causation: The plaintiff's illness or injury is directly caused by the defendant's negligent breach of duty.

21. C: A testifying expert with conflict of interest should be ruled out as quickly as possible without divulging the primary content of the case, so the information that should be shared is the names of the parties involved, significant players and facilities that may be involved but are not currently parties to the action, and any insurance companies involved. Conflicts can occur if the TE has or has had a relationship with any party to the suit or if a family member or close associate has such a relationship.

22. B: In most cases, a consulting expert's notes and opinions, especially regarding strengths and weaknesses of a case, are not discoverable since they are considered work products of the attorney and thereby protected; however, if a testifying expert utilizes the consulting expert's opinions and notes in order to form an opinion, then this opens them to discovery. Notes and opinions may also be discoverable if the consulting expert is the sole expert on the subject or other experts would be unable to carry out the same examination.

23. A: A products liability case involves those who manufacture and sell products and can include not only buyers but also those who use or are exposed to the product. Categories include medical devices (such as implants) and drugs (including severe adverse reactions), non-medical devices (such as automobiles, food, and consumer and industrial products). Exposure to hazardous chemicals in the workplace is an environmental case. Physician delay of treatment is medical malpractice. Failure of insurance company to pay claims is a case in which health is an issue.

Copyright © Mometrix Media. You have been licensed one copy of this document for personal use only. Any other reproduction or redistribution is strictly prohibited. All rights reserved.

24. C: Interrogatory: A list of questions is sent from one party to a second party requesting that the second party respond under oath in writing. Deposition: Person asked questions under oath with a court reporter present and recording the proceedings. Request for production of documents: Request for specific documents (such as bank statements). Request for admission: A request is sent from one party to a second party that the second party admits to specific facts.

25. C: Administering a blood product to a Jehovah Witness despite the patient's explicit refusal is an example of an intentional tort because the physician, the tortfeasor (wrongdoer) carried out the act with intention, ignoring the patient's refusal while understanding that it might cause the patient emotional stress. This type of intentional tort may be considered an act of battery by the physician even though the underlying intent may have been to save the patient's life.

26. B: While all of these are important, the CLNC should focus on the weaknesses of the case, as this may be the primary factor for the attorney deciding whether or not to take a case, especially since the attorney may not receive any compensation if the case is too weak to win. Strengths and extent of injury are also important. For example, pursuing a case for minor injuries may not be cost-effective. Availability of testifying experts is a concern but less so during the initial screening.

27. D: Mediation: Involves both parties to a dispute sitting down with a third party to try to work out a voluntary settlement. Arbitration: Allowing a third party to hear a dispute at a formal hearing after which the third party makes an award or decision. Mini-trial: Attorneys present abbreviated cases to a neutral party or advisory jury selected from both parties to the dispute. The opinion is nonbinding. Summary jury trial: Attorneys present abbreviated cases to a jury (selected from the jury pool), which renders a nonbinding advisory judgment.

28. C: A toxic tort involves chemical exposure that results in the person's injury or disease. Toxic torts may arise from consumer-product exposure, such as the formaldehyde-treated carpet; occupational exposure, such as from industrial chemicals or pesticides; and pharmaceuticals, such as a drug that caused unexpected adverse effects (often to large numbers of people). Toxic substances frequently implicated in toxic tort cases include asbestos, pesticides, silica, and benzene. Toxic exposure may occur directly (such as from being sprayed with pesticides or taking of medications) or indirectly (such as from drinking contaminated groundwater).

29. A: Any mismatch of ink or pressure of writing may indicate that tampering of the medical record has occurred. Other signs of tampering include erasures, words obliterated or crossed out so they are unreadable, crowding of entries, and differences in handwriting, such as different slant to writing, or too much uniformity, which may indicate an attempt to copy someone's handwriting. Incident reports, films, MRI films, and billing statements must be requested separately as they are not part of the medical record.

Copyright © Mometrix Media. You have been licensed one copy of this document for personal use only. Any other reproduction or redistribution is strictly prohibited. All rights reserved.

30. D: Reports should be written so that they can be scanned and read rapidly and easily understood, so definitions should be included in the body of the report, usually in parentheses after the medical term, so that the reader does not need to look elsewhere for information. Definitions should be simple and should cover medical terms as well as abbreviations. The CNLC should anticipate the questions that might arise and attempt to address those issues in the report.

31. B: *Respondeat superior:* An employer is considered directly responsible for negligence of its employees toward clients. Ostensible liability: An employer is responsible for negligence of independent contractors employed as agents for the employer. Direct corporate liability: A corporation has legal responsibilities and is responsible for negligent acts of the corporation and its agents. Employer's liability: This is not a form of vicarious liability but is direct responsibility for negligent acts of an employer toward employees.

32. A: The most likely case to be rejected would be the 80-year-old patient who suffered postoperative complications but recovered fully. Generally, attorneys are less likely to pursue cases that involve very elderly patients or cases in which the patient recovered fully or had no physical injury, as these types of cases are more difficult to prove causation and negligence. Plaintiff attorneys are usually most concerned with taking cases that they can win and that are economically viable.

33. C: The American Board of Forensic Document Examiners (ABFDE) provides the only certification for FDEs and sets minimum requirements for certification: Baccalaureate degree, participation in a full-time training program in a recognized legitimate document laboratory, and working in a full-time FDE practice. Graphologists are often self-trained or have taken online or correspondence courses and may vary widely in skill levels and training. Experience alone is not adequate, since many unqualified practitioners of graphology have testified in court.

34. D: In a state in which the tort of intentional spoliation (intentional destruction of evidence) is not recognized, the purpose of presenting evidence that the destruction occurred is to sway the jury to believe that the defendant is shielding himself or herself from damaging evidence and to thereby strengthen the case for the plaintiff. Most states do not recognize intentional spoliation at this time and, therefore, no legal action is taken toward defendants who destroy or "lose" evidence, but the CNLC should note any indication that this has occurred.

35. C: Because experts in any field tend to be high profile and to publish findings or be referenced in other authors' articles, the best way to identify an expert is to begin by searching for the particular topic/disorder in an online database, such as MEDLINE, and to note which authors' names have multiple entries. Once a potential expert is noted, then the author's articles can be accessed online. Most journals provide archives of older articles as well as current, and the author's published material should be evaluated thoroughly prior to contacting the person.

Copyright © Mometrix Media. You have been licensed one copy of this document for personal use only. Any other reproduction or redistribution is strictly prohibited. All rights reserved.

36. A: If standards of care were not adhered to and the defense can't prove otherwise, then the defense must attempt to show the reason. In this case, since an innovative treatment was utilized, the best defense may be that the standards don't yet reflect current cutting-edge medical treatments. In many cases, new treatment protocols and procedures occur more frequently than changes to standards of care. Other arguments can include that SOC don't apply, are too general to quantify, or the SOC cited doesn't apply to the current case.

37. B: There are three types of utilization review: prospective (which assesses the need for care prior to treatment), concurrent (which assesses the need for continued care while the patient is being treated), and retrospective (which reviews the medical necessity and efficacy of treatment already provided). Prospective utilization review has the highest potential for liability because it is at this point that medical care may be denied or limited in some way. Concurrent utilization review can also have high potential for liability if it results in too early discontinuation of treatment. Retrospective review has the lowest potential for liability.

38. D: NCQA has 5 levels of accreditation: full accreditation, accreditation with recommendations, one-year accreditation, provisional accreditation, and denial or revocation of accreditation. NCQA accredits MCOs, such as HMOs that have been operating for at least 18 months and have comprehensive health care services available to specific populations. NCQA also has 6 categories of standards that it reviews as part of accreditation: quality improvement, utilization management, physician credentialing, members' rights and responsibilities, preventive services, and medical records/peer review.

39. C: Requests for production directed to plaintiffs include:
General: Product alleged to cause injury, police reports, diaries, photos, videos, employment records.
Medical: Medical records and authorizations.
Witnesses: Reports, documents, other demonstrative evidence to be used by or prepared by the testifying expert.
Financial: Medical bills, tax returns, financial statements, and withholding forms.
The request for production should include the date by which the items should be produced and should include specific instructions about each item requested. Plaintiffs may respond and indicate if items are not in their possession or if they object to producing items.

40. D: Financial request for production directed to defendants would likely include insurance policies, documents regarding the financial status of the facility, and any incentive compensation plans. Medical bills, tax returns, and withholding forms would likely be directed to plaintiffs. The plaintiff would likely ask the defendant for all documents referred to in interrogatories or documents that will be referred to during the court proceedings. Requests may be quite extensive since the plaintiffs and their representatives may not know in advance which evidence is significant.

Copyright © Mometrix Media. You have been licensed one copy of this document for personal use only. Any other reproduction or redistribution is strictly prohibited. All rights reserved.

41. C: Because this accident involved moving violations, the best medium is that which reconstructs the events, the computer-generated animation, since this helps the jurors to visualize and understand the accident and how the plaintiff received injuries. Photos are inexpensive but static and show only a moment in time, not the chain of events. A recording can show only the distress of the caller, which might help sway a jury, but it doesn't show how the accident occurred. Hand-drawn illustrations are usually more crudely drawn and less impressive to a jury.

42. D: The CLNC should deliver the materials, assuming that the testifying expert will be able to identify necessary information. Under no circumstances should the documents be altered by underlining or highlighting because this may make it seem as though the expert has been coached. The CLNC should not provide any written documents to guide the testifying expert, as these may be discoverable. The testifying expert is expected to testify on the facts of the case in an unbiased manner.

43. B: Testifying experts are often considered biased by jurors, especially since experts for the plaintiff and the defense may contradict each other, so the best response is to say, "I don't take every case, just those I believe have merit" to counter the claim that the fee is the primary motivation for testifying. Opposing attorneys often ask about the TE's fee, percentage of income derived for serving as a TE, and whether the TE has a financial interest in the outcome of the case to establish bias.

44. A: A practicing neurosurgeon would be able to testify with expertise about the condition based on academic preparation as well as clinical experience. Medical experts have better credibility if they are currently working in the field more than 50% of the time, since those who are retired or serve only as expert witnesses may be looked upon as "hired guns" whose primary concern is income. Experts should be board-certified in the field in which they are testifying. Nurses do not testify about medical diagnoses, only nursing diagnoses.

45. D: A contract usually begins with an introduction, a preamble, and a statement of agreement. The body contains a number of different clauses, generally beginning with the definitions, in which the consulting services that the CLNC is to provide would be outlined. However, the consideration clause outlines the fee to be paid in exchange for services. Consideration may be monetary or non-monetary (such as an exchange for services rather than a fee), but contracts are usually considered invalid without some type of consideration for services.

46. B: Prior to signing a contract with a client, the CLNC should hire an attorney who specializes in contracts to review the contract, since contract language can be quite complicated and inconsistencies may be present. The attorney should especially review those clauses that may pose problems, such as consideration, duration of the agreement, tax liability, indemnification, issues of confidentiality, non-competition, conflicts of interest, delegation, time of the essence, and arbitration.

Copyright © Mometrix Media. You have been licensed one copy of this document for personal use only. Any other reproduction or redistribution is strictly prohibited. All rights reserved.

47. C: Substantial factor. Causation in fact (actual causation in which the defendant is the cause of damages) is determined by two different tests:

But for: The damages would not have occurred but for the actions of the defendant.

Substantial factor: The actions of the defendant were a substantial factor in the damages even though other factors may have also been involved.

Another issue in causation is foreseeability, or the idea that the defendant should have foreseen that certain actions, such as failure to complete work on time, would result in damages.

48. B: The CLNC cannot advise clients about the statute of limitations because this is providing legal advice. The CLNC can facilitate the communication between client and attorney, such as by preparing a list of client questions, and can communicate the response but cannot interpret or elaborate on the response. The CLNC cannot advise clients about the merits of a case or advise them whether or not they should settle a case. Additionally the CLNC should not carry out any independent investigations for the client or prepare any legal documents for any client unless under the supervision or direction of an attorney.

49. A: The CLNC should prepare an interview script but should learn the material thoroughly and avoid memorization because the interview is guided by the potential client, who may veer in different directions from the script. Additionally, a memorized presentation often sounds memorized, and that can be a barrier to communication. The CLNC should not subject the potential client to video, PowerPoint or other types of electronic presentations during an interview and should avoid using notes, which suggest the CLNC is not prepared.

50. A: The purpose of requesting certified medical records is to ensure that the records have been reviewed and certified as complete by the administrator of records. This does not mean, however, that all patient records or products are included as different departments, such as the cardiac catheterization lab, may maintain separate records and products, such as ECG strips, which are not included in the regular medical records, so further discovery may be necessary. Ensuring that records are complete does not ensure there have been no alterations.

Copyright © Mometrix Media. You have been licensed one copy of this document for personal use only. Any other reproduction or redistribution is strictly prohibited. All rights reserved.

Secret Key #1 – Time is Your Greatest Enemy

Pace Yourself

Wear a watch to the LEGAL NURSE Test. At the beginning of the test, check the time (or start a chronometer on your watch to count the minutes), and check the time after each passage or every few questions to make sure you are "on schedule." For the computerized test an onscreen clock display will keep track of your remaining time, but it may be easier for you to monitor your pace based on how many minutes have been used, rather than how many minutes remain.

If you are forced to speed up, do it efficiently. Usually one or more answer choices can be eliminated without too much difficulty. Above all, don't panic. Don't speed up and just begin guessing at random choices. By pacing yourself, and continually monitoring your progress against the clock or your watch, you will always know exactly how far ahead or behind you are with your available time. If you find that you are one minute behind on the test, don't skip one question without spending any time on it, just to catch back up. Spend perhaps 45 seconds on the question and after four questions, you will have caught back up more gradually. Once you catch back up, you can continue working each problem at your normal pace.

Furthermore, don't dwell on the problems that you were rushed on. If a problem was taking up too much time and you made a hurried guess, it must be difficult. The difficult questions are the ones you are most likely to miss anyway, so it isn't a big loss. It is better to end with more time than you need than to run out of time. You can always go back and work the problems that you skipped. If you have time left over, as you review the skipped questions, start at the earliest skipped question, spend at most another minute, and then move on to the next skipped question.

Lastly, sometimes it is beneficial to slow down if you are constantly getting ahead of time. You are always more likely to catch a careless mistake by working more slowly than quickly, and among very high-scoring test takers (those who are likely to have lots of time left over), careless errors affect the score more than mastery of material.

Copyright © Mometrix Media. You have been licensed one copy of this document for personal use only. Any other reproduction or redistribution is strictly prohibited. All rights reserved.

The table below shows the breakdown of the exam.
- Initiating the Project
- Planning the Project
- Executing the Project
- Controlling the Project
- Closing the Project
- Professional Responsibility

200 multiple choice questions – 4 hours on the computer
15 minute prep tutorial.

Secret Key #2 – Guessing is not Guesswork

You probably know that guessing is a good idea on the LEGAL NURSE test- unlike other standardized tests, there is no penalty for getting a wrong answer. Even if you have no idea about a question, you still have a 20-25% chance of getting it right.

Most test takers do not understand the impact that proper guessing can have on their score. Unless you score extremely high, guessing will significantly contribute to your final score.

Monkeys Take the LEGAL NURSE

What most test takers don't realize is that to insure that 20-25% chance, you have to guess randomly. If you put 20 monkeys in a room to take this test, assuming they answered once per question and behaved themselves, on average they would get 20-25% of the questions correct. Put 20 test takers in the room, and the average will be much lower among guessed questions. Why?

- This test intentionally writes deceptive answer choices that "look" right. A test taker has no idea about a question, so picks the "best looking" answer, which is often

Copyright © Mometrix Media. You have been licensed one copy of this document for personal use only. Any other reproduction or redistribution is strictly prohibited. All rights reserved.

wrong. The monkey has no idea what looks good and what doesn't, so will consistently be lucky about 20-25% of the time.

- Test takers will eliminate answer choices from the guessing pool based on a hunch or intuition. Simple but correct answers often get excluded, leaving a 0% chance of being correct. The monkey has no clue, and often gets lucky with the best choice.

This is why the process of elimination endorsed by most test courses is flawed and detrimental to your performance- test takers don't guess, they make an ignorant stab in the dark that is usually worse than random.

Success Strategy #2

Let me introduce one of the most valuable ideas of this course- the $5 challenge:

You only mark your "best guess" if you are willing to bet $5 on it.
You only eliminate choices from guessing if you are willing to bet $5 on it.

Why $5? Five dollars is an amount of money that is small yet not insignificant, and can really add up fast (20 questions could cost you $100). Likewise, each answer choice on one question of the LEGAL NURSE will have a small impact on your overall score, but it can really add up to a lot of points in the end.

The process of elimination IS valuable. The following shows your chance of guessing it right:

If you eliminate this many choices:	0	1	2	3	4
Chance of getting it correct	20%	25%	33%	50%	100%

However, if you accidentally eliminate the right answer or go on a hunch for an incorrect answer, your chances drop dramatically: to 0%. By guessing among all the answer choices, you are GUARANTEED to have a shot at the right answer.

That's why the $5 test is so valuable- if you give up the advantage and safety of a pure guess, it had better be worth the risk.

Copyright © Mometrix Media. You have been licensed one copy of this document for personal use only.
Any other reproduction or redistribution is strictly prohibited. All rights reserved.

What we still haven't covered is how to be sure that whatever guess you make is truly random. Here's the easiest way:

Always pick the first answer choice among those remaining.

Such a technique means that you have decided, **before you see a single test question**, exactly how you are going to guess- and since the order of choices tells you nothing about which one is correct, this guessing technique is perfectly random.

Secret Key #3 – Practice Smarter, Not Harder

Many test takers delay the test preparation process because they dread the awful amounts of practice time they think necessary to succeed on the test. We have refined an effective method that will take you only a fraction of the time.

There are a number of "obstacles" in your way on the LEGAL NURSE test. Among these are answering questions, finishing in time, and mastering test-taking strategies. All must be executed on the day of the test at peak performance, or your score will suffer. The LEGAL NURSE is a mental marathon that has a large impact on your future.

Just like a marathon runner, it is important to work your way up to the full challenge. So first you just worry about questions, and then time, and finally strategy:

Success Strategy

1. Find a good source for practice tests.
2. If you are willing to make a larger time investment, consider using more than one study guide- often the different approaches of multiple authors will help you "get" difficult concepts.
3. Take a practice test with no time constraints, with all study helps "open book." Take your time with questions and focus on applying strategies.

Copyright © Mometrix Media. You have been licensed one copy of this document for personal use only.
Any other reproduction or redistribution is strictly prohibited. All rights reserved.

4. Take a practice test with time constraints, with all guides "open book."

5. Take a final practice test with no open material and time limits

If you have time to take more practice tests, just repeat step 5. By gradually exposing yourself to the full rigors of the test environment, you will condition your mind to the stress of test day and maximize your success.

Secret Key #4 - Prepare, Don't Procrastinate

Let me state an obvious fact: if you take the test three times, you will get three different scores. This is due to the way you feel on test day, the level of preparedness you have, and, despite the test writers' claims to the contrary, some tests WILL be easier for you than others.

Since your future depends so much on your score, you should maximize your chances of success. In order to maximize the likelihood of success, you've got to prepare in advance. This means taking practice tests and spending time learning the information and test taking strategies you will need to succeed.

Never take the test as a "practice" test, expecting that you can just take it again if you need to. Feel free to take sample tests on your own, but when you go to take the official test, be prepared, be focused, and do your best the first time!

Secret Key #5 - Test Yourself

Everyone knows that time is money. There is no need to spend too much of your time or too little of your time preparing for the test. You should only spend as much of your precious time preparing as is necessary for you to get the score you need.

Once you have taken a practice test under real conditions of time constraints, then you will know if you are ready for the test or not.

Copyright © Mometrix Media. You have been licensed one copy of this document for personal use only. Any other reproduction or redistribution is strictly prohibited. All rights reserved.

If you have scored extremely high the first time that you take the practice test, then there is not much point in spending countless hours studying. You are already there.

Benchmark your abilities by retaking practice tests and seeing how much you have improved. Once you score high enough to guarantee success, then you are ready.

If you have scored well below where you need, then knuckle down and begin studying in earnest. Check your improvement regularly through the use of practice tests under real conditions. Above all, don't worry, panic, or give up. The key is perseverance!

Then, when you go to take the test, remain confident and remember how well you did on the practice tests. If you can score high enough on a practice test, then you can do the same on the real thing.

Copyright © Mometrix Media. You have been licensed one copy of this document for personal use only. Any other reproduction or redistribution is strictly prohibited. All rights reserved.

General Strategies

The most important thing you can do is to ignore your fears and jump into the test immediately- do not be overwhelmed by any strange-sounding terms. You have to jump into the test like jumping into a pool- all at once is the easiest way.

Make Predictions

As you read and understand the question, try to guess what the answer will be. Remember that several of the answer choices are wrong, and once you begin reading them, your mind will immediately become cluttered with answer choices designed to throw you off. Your mind is typically the most focused immediately after you have read the question and digested its contents. If you can, try to predict what the correct answer will be. You may be surprised at what you can predict.

Quickly scan the choices and see if your prediction is in the listed answer choices. If it is, then you can be quite confident that you have the right answer. It still won't hurt to check the other answer choices, but most of the time, you've got it!

Answer the Question

It may seem obvious to only pick answer choices that answer the question, but the test writers can create some excellent answer choices that are wrong. Don't pick an answer just because it sounds right, or you believe it to be true. It MUST answer the question. Once you've made your selection, always go back and check it against the question and make sure that you didn't misread the question, and the answer choice does answer the question posed.

Benchmark

After you read the first answer choice, decide if you think it sounds correct or not. If it doesn't, move on to the next answer choice. If it does, mentally mark that answer choice. This doesn't mean that you've definitely selected it as your answer choice, it just means

Copyright © Mometrix Media. You have been licensed one copy of this document for personal use only. Any other reproduction or redistribution is strictly prohibited. All rights reserved.

that it's the best you've seen thus far. Go ahead and read the next choice. If the next choice is worse than the one you've already selected, keep going to the next answer choice. If the next choice is better than the choice you've already selected, mentally mark the new answer choice as your best guess.

The first answer choice that you select becomes your standard. Every other answer choice must be benchmarked against that standard. That choice is correct until proven otherwise by another answer choice beating it out. Once you've decided that no other answer choice seems as good, do one final check to ensure that your answer choice answers the question posed.

Valid Information

Don't discount any of the information provided in the question. Every piece of information may be necessary to determine the correct answer. None of the information in the question is there to throw you off (while the answer choices will certainly have information to throw you off). If two seemingly unrelated topics are discussed, don't ignore either. You can be confident there is a relationship, or it wouldn't be included in the question, and you are probably going to have to determine what is that relationship to find the answer.

Avoid "Fact Traps"

Don't get distracted by a choice that is factually true. Your search is for the answer that answers the question. Stay focused and don't fall for an answer that is true but incorrect. Always go back to the question and make sure you're choosing an answer that actually answers the question and is not just a true statement. An answer can be factually correct, but it MUST answer the question asked. Additionally, two answers can both be seemingly correct, so be sure to read all of the answer choices, and make sure that you get the one that BEST answers the question.

Milk the Question

Some of the questions may throw you completely off. They might deal with a subject you have not been exposed to, or one that you haven't reviewed in years. While your lack of knowledge about the subject will be a hindrance, the question itself can give you many

Copyright © Mometrix Media. You have been licensed one copy of this document for personal use only. Any other reproduction or redistribution is strictly prohibited. All rights reserved.

clues that will help you find the correct answer. Read the question carefully and look for clues. Watch particularly for adjectives and nouns describing difficult terms or words that you don't recognize. Regardless of if you completely understand a word or not, replacing it with a synonym either provided or one you more familiar with may help you to understand what the questions are asking. Rather than wracking your mind about specific detailed information concerning a difficult term or word, try to use mental substitutes that are easier to understand.

The Trap of Familiarity

Don't just choose a word because you recognize it. On difficult questions, you may not recognize a number of words in the answer choices. The test writers don't put "make-believe" words on the test; so don't think that just because you only recognize all the words in one answer choice means that answer choice must be correct. If you only recognize words in one answer choice, then focus on that one. Is it correct? Try your best to determine if it is correct. If it is, that is great, but if it doesn't, eliminate it. Each word and answer choice you eliminate increases your chances of getting the question correct, even if you then have to guess among the unfamiliar choices.

Eliminate Answers

Eliminate choices as soon as you realize they are wrong. But be careful! Make sure you consider all of the possible answer choices. Just because one appears right, doesn't mean that the next one won't be even better! The test writers will usually put more than one good answer choice for every question, so read all of them. Don't worry if you are stuck between two that seem right. By getting down to just two remaining possible choices, your odds are now 50/50. Rather than wasting too much time, play the odds. You are guessing, but guessing wisely, because you've been able to knock out some of the answer choices that you know are wrong. If you are eliminating choices and realize that the last answer choice you are left with is also obviously wrong, don't panic. Start over and consider each choice again. There may easily be something that you missed the first time and will realize on the second pass.

Copyright © Mometrix Media. You have been licensed one copy of this document for personal use only. Any other reproduction or redistribution is strictly prohibited. All rights reserved.

Tough Questions

If you are stumped on a problem or it appears too hard or too difficult, don't waste time. Move on! Remember though, if you can quickly check for obviously incorrect answer choices, your chances of guessing correctly are greatly improved. Before you completely give up, at least try to knock out a couple of possible answers. Eliminate what you can and then guess at the remaining answer choices before moving on.

Brainstorm

If you get stuck on a difficult question, spend a few seconds quickly brainstorming. Run through the complete list of possible answer choices. Look at each choice and ask yourself, "Could this answer the question satisfactorily?" Go through each answer choice and consider it independently of the other. By systematically going through all possibilities, you may find something that you would otherwise overlook. Remember that when you get stuck, it's important to try to keep moving.

Read Carefully

Understand the problem. Read the question and answer choices carefully. Don't miss the question because you misread the terms. You have plenty of time to read each question thoroughly and make sure you understand what is being asked. Yet a happy medium must be attained, so don't waste too much time. You must read carefully, but efficiently.

Face Value

When in doubt, use common sense. Always accept the situation in the problem at face value. Don't read too much into it. These problems will not require you to make huge leaps of logic. The test writers aren't trying to throw you off with a cheap trick. If you have to go beyond creativity and make a leap of logic in order to have an answer choice answer the question, then you should look at the other answer choices. Don't overcomplicate the problem by creating theoretical relationships or explanations that will warp time or space. These are normal problems rooted in reality. It's just that the applicable relationship or explanation may not be readily apparent and you have to figure things out. Use your common sense to interpret anything that isn't clear.

Copyright © Mometrix Media. You have been licensed one copy of this document for personal use only. Any other reproduction or redistribution is strictly prohibited. All rights reserved.

Prefixes

If you're having trouble with a word in the question or answer choices, try dissecting it. Take advantage of every clue that the word might include. Prefixes and suffixes can be a huge help. Usually they allow you to determine a basic meaning. Pre- means before, post-means after, pro - is positive, de- is negative. From these prefixes and suffixes, you can get an idea of the general meaning of the word and try to put it into context. Beware though of any traps. Just because con is the opposite of pro, doesn't necessarily mean congress is the opposite of progress!

Hedge Phrases

Watch out for critical "hedge" phrases, such as likely, may, can, will often, sometimes, often, almost, mostly, usually, generally, rarely, sometimes. Question writers insert these hedge phrases to cover every possibility. Often an answer choice will be wrong simply because it leaves no room for exception. Avoid answer choices that have definitive words like "exactly," and "always".

Switchback Words

Stay alert for "switchbacks". These are the words and phrases frequently used to alert you to shifts in thought. The most common switchback word is "but". Others include although, however, nevertheless, on the other hand, even though, while, in spite of, despite, regardless of.

New Information

Correct answer choices will rarely have completely new information included. Answer choices typically are straightforward reflections of the material asked about and will directly relate to the question. If a new piece of information is included in an answer choice that doesn't even seem to relate to the topic being asked about, then that answer choice is likely incorrect. All of the information needed to answer the question is usually provided for you, and so you should not have to make guesses that are unsupported or choose answer choices that require unknown information that cannot be reasoned on its own.

Copyright © Mometrix Media. You have been licensed one copy of this document for personal use only. Any other reproduction or redistribution is strictly prohibited. All rights reserved.

Time Management

On technical questions, don't get lost on the technical terms. Don't spend too much time on any one question. If you don't know what a term means, then since you don't have a dictionary, odds are you aren't going to get much further. You should immediately recognize terms as whether or not you know them. If you don't, work with the other clues that you have, the other answer choices and terms provided, but don't waste too much time trying to figure out a difficult term.

Contextual Clues

Look for contextual clues. An answer can be right but not correct. The contextual clues will help you find the answer that is most right and is correct. Understand the context in which a phrase or statement is made. This will help you make important distinctions.

Don't Panic

Panicking will not answer any questions for you. Therefore, it isn't helpful. When you first see the question, if your mind goes blank, take a deep breath. Force yourself to mechanically go through the steps of solving the problem and using the strategies you've learned.

Pace Yourself

Don't get clock fever. It's easy to be overwhelmed when you're looking at a page full of questions, your mind is full of random thoughts and feeling confused, and the clock is ticking down faster than you would like. Calm down and maintain the pace that you have set for yourself. As long as you are on track by monitoring your pace, you are guaranteed to have enough time for yourself. When you get to the last few minutes of the test, it may seem like you won't have enough time left, but if you only have as many questions as you should have left at that point, then you're right on track!

Copyright © Mometrix Media. You have been licensed one copy of this document for personal use only. Any other reproduction or redistribution is strictly prohibited. All rights reserved.

Answer Selection

The best way to pick an answer choice is to eliminate all of those that are wrong, until only one is left and confirm that is the correct answer. Sometimes though, an answer choice may immediately look right. Be careful! Take a second to make sure that the other choices are not equally obvious. Don't make a hasty mistake. There are only two times that you should stop before checking other answers. First is when you are positive that the answer choice you have selected is correct. Second is when time is almost out and you have to make a quick guess!

Check Your Work

Since you will probably not know every term listed and the answer to every question, it is important that you get credit for the ones that you do know. Don't miss any questions through careless mistakes. If at all possible, try to take a second to look back over your answer selection and make sure you've selected the correct answer choice and haven't made a costly careless mistake (such as marking an answer choice that you didn't mean to mark). This quick double check should more than pay for itself in caught mistakes for the time it costs.

Beware of Directly Quoted Answers

Sometimes an answer choice will repeat word for word a portion of the question or reference section. However, beware of such exact duplication – it may be a trap! More than likely, the correct choice will paraphrase or summarize a point, rather than being exactly the same wording.

Slang

Scientific sounding answers are better than slang ones. An answer choice that begins "To compare the outcomes..." is much more likely to be correct than one that begins "Because some people insisted..."

Copyright © Mometrix Media. You have been licensed one copy of this document for personal use only. Any other reproduction or redistribution is strictly prohibited. All rights reserved.

Extreme Statements

Avoid wild answers that throw out highly controversial ideas that are proclaimed as established fact. An answer choice that states the "process should be used in certain situations, if…" is much more likely to be correct than one that states the "process should be discontinued completely." The first is a calm rational statement and doesn't even make a definitive, uncompromising stance, using a hedge word "if" to provide wiggle room, whereas the second choice is a radical idea and far more extreme.

Answer Choice Families

When you have two or more answer choices that are direct opposites or parallels, one of them is usually the correct answer. For instance, if one answer choice states "x increases" and another answer choice states "x decreases" or "y increases," then those two or three answer choices are very similar in construction and fall into the same family of answer choices. A family of answer choices is when two or three answer choices are very similar in construction, and yet often have a directly opposite meaning. Usually the correct answer choice will be in that family of answer choices. The "odd man out" or answer choice that doesn't seem to fit the parallel construction of the other answer choices is more likely to be incorrect.

Copyright © Mometrix Media. You have been licensed one copy of this document for personal use only. Any other reproduction or redistribution is strictly prohibited. All rights reserved.

Special Report: Additional Bonus Material

Due to our efforts to try to keep this book to a manageable length, we've created a link that will give you access to all of your additional bonus material.

Please visit http://www.mometrix.com/bonus948/clnc to access the information.

Copyright © Mometrix Media. You have been licensed one copy of this document for personal use only. Any other reproduction or redistribution is strictly prohibited. All rights reserved.